D1555780

# Revision Hip Arthroplasty

# Revision Hip Arthroplasty:
## A Practical Approach to Bone Stock Loss

Edited by

**Richard N. Villar**, BSc, MS, FRCS
Consultant Orthopaedic Surgeon, Addenbrooke's Hospital, Cambridge, UK

**Allan E. Gross**, MD, FRCS (C)
Head, Division of Orthopaedic Surgery, Mount Sinai Hospital; Professor of Surgery, University of Toronto, Canada

**Derek McMinn**, MB, BS, FRCS
Consultant Orthopaedic Surgeon, Midland International Orthopaedic Service, Birmingham Nuffield Hospital, Birmingham, UK

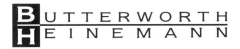
BUTTERWORTH
HEINEMANN

Butterworth-Heinemann
Linacre House, Jordan Hill, Oxford OX2 8DP
A division of Reed Educational and Professional Publishing Ltd

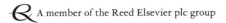 A member of the Reed Elsevier plc group

OXFORD  BOSTON  JOHANNESBURG
MELBOURNE  NEW DELHI  SINGAPORE

First published 1997

British Library Cataloguing in Publication Data

Revision hip arthroplasty: a practical approach to bone
   stock loss
   1   Total hip replacement      2   Hip – Reoperation
   I   Villar, Richard N.      II   Gross, Allan E.      III   McMinn, Derek
   617.5'81'059

ISBN 0 7506 1640 7

Library of Congress Cataloguing in Publication Data
Revision hip arthroplasty: a practical approach to bone stock loss/
   edited by Richard N. Villar, Allan E. Gross, and Derek McMinn.
   p.     cm
   Includes bibliographical references and index.
   ISBN 0 7506 1640 7
   1   Total hip replacement – Reoperation.      I   Villar, Richard N.
   II Gross, Allan E.      III   McMinn, Derek.
   [DNLM: 1   Hip Joint – Surgery      2   Hip Prosthesis.      3   Reoperation –
   methods.      4   Arthroplasty.      5   Osteolysis – surgery.      WE 860 R453
   RD549.R425
   617.5'810592–dc20
                                                              96–9042
                                                              CIP

Printed and bound in Great Britain at The Bath Press plc, Bath

# Contents

# Contributors

**Michael M. Alexiades**, MD
Assistant Professor of Orthopaedic Surgery,
Cornell University Medical College; Attendant,
Lenox Hill Hospital and Hospital for Special
Surgery, New York, USA

**Timothy M. Bull**, FRCS
Senior Registrar, Addenbrooke's Hospital,
Cambridge, UK

**Pieter Buma**, PhD
Biologist, Institute of Orthopaedics, University
Hospital, Nijmegen, The Netherlands

**Robert W. Eberle**
Independent Consultant, Clinical Information
Consultants Inc., Columbus, Ohio, USA

**Jean Gardeniers**, MD, PhD
Orthopaedic Surgeon, Institute of Orthopaedics,
University Hospital, Nijmegen, The Netherlands

**Allan E. Gross**, MD FRCS(C)
Head, Division of Orthopaedic Surgery, Mount
Sinai Hospital; Professor, Department of
Surgery, University of Toronto, Canada

**Kevin Hardinge**, M. Ch. Orth, FRCS
Consultant Orthopaedic Surgeon, Wrightington
Hospital for Joint Diseases; Hunterian Professor,
Royal College of Surgeons of England

**Donald W. Howie**, MB, BS, PhD, FAOrthA,
FRACS
Professor of Orthopaedic Surgery and Trauma,
University of Adelaide; Head of Department of
Orthopaedic Surgery and Trauma, Royal
Adelaide Hospital, Australia

**Rik Huiskes**, PhD
Professor of Biomechanics, University of
Nijmegen, The Netherlands

**Graham S. Keene**, FRCS(Orth), MB, BS
Senior Orthopaedic Registrar, Addenbrooke's
Hospital, Cambridge, UK

**Thomas H. Mallory**, MD, FACS
Chairman of Joint Implant Surgery Section,
Grant Medical Center, Columbus, Ohio;
Clinical Assistant Professor, Orthopaedic
Surgery, Ohio State University, Columbus,
Ohio, USA

**Derek McMinn**, MB, BS, FRCS
Consultant Orthopaedic Surgeon, Midland
International Orthopaedic Service, Birmingham
Nuffield Hospital, Birmingham, UK

**Maria B. Mitchell**
Clinical Research Coordinator, Grant
Orthopaedic Institute, Columbus, Ohio, USA

**S. Ranawat**, MD
Director, Department of Orthopaedics and Center
for Total Joint Replacement at Lenox Hill
Hospital, New York, USA

**Bruce H. Robie**, PhD
Assistant Director for Design and Production
Department of Biomechanics and Biomaterials,
Hospital for Special Surgery, New York, USA

**Jose A. Rodriguez**, MD
Clinical Instructor, Cornell University Medical
College; attending Surgeon Lenox Hill Hospital
and Hospital for Special Surgery, New York,
USA

**Jan Willem Schimmel**
Orthopaedic Surgeon, Leeuwarden Medical
Centre, The Netherlands

**B. Willem Schreurs**, MD, PhD
Orthopaedic Surgeon, Institute of Orthopaedics,
University Hospital of Nijmegen, The Netherlands

**Tom J.J.H. Slooff**, MD, PhD
Professor of Orthopaedics, Institute of
Orthopaedics, University Hospital of Nijmegen,
The Netherlands

**Ian Stockley**, MD, FRCS
Consultant Orthopaedic Surgeon, Northern
General Hospital, Sheffield, UK

**Richard N. Villar**, BSc, MS, FRCS
Consultant Orthopaedic Surgeon, Addenbrooke's
Hospital; Clinical Director, Cambridge Hip and
Knee Unit, Cambridge, UK

**Timothy M. Wright**, PhD
Director, Department of Biomechanics and
Biomaterials, Hospital for Special Surgery, New
York, USA

# Preface

It seemed such a simple idea at the time. Why not write a book on bone stock loss in revision hip surgery? But once one starts, only then comes the realization of the enormous efforts required of such a task.

This book was born out of the various British courses in revision surgery that have taken place over the years, latterly in Stratford-upon-Avon, England. Gathered there have been some of the world's most influential names in the subspecialty, many of whom have taken the time and trouble to contribute to this book. We cannot pretend that the text covers every aspect of bone stock loss management but trust it considers those angles that the practising orthopaedic surgeon would wish to know. All who have written these pages are hard-working, frontline, orthopaedic surgeons. Each of us is familiar with the successes, failures, and even disasters that revision operations can bring.

Revision surgery is here to stay. As the numbers of primary replacements rise, as the demands of patients increase, so there comes a greater requirement for revision operations. In the ideal world, perhaps, all revisions should be performed by specialists in the field. Life is not so simple. The problems of bone loss can now face any orthopaedic surgeon, at any time. It is not always possible or practical to refer the patient on elsewhere. We now realize that there are no shortcuts in revision surgery. Its techniques are demanding, its equipment expensive. No longer can it be left as a procedure for the most junior trainee to undertake, away from the guiding hand of his chief. The fact that a primary replacement has failed does not mean that the patient should be denied the best effort at reconstruction.

Bone grafting is now big business and within these pages may be found a variety of different approaches to the problem. Some believe in massive grafts, others in morsellized, while a number consider it should not be used at all. We fear it must be the reader's task to decide which approach is best. All we can do is to tell you of our own experiences in the hope that your decision-making will be easier. Welcome to an insoluble problem that we, as editors, have tried to unravel.

R.N.V.
A.E.G.
D.M.

# Acknowledgements

It may not appear large, but this book took much effort to edit and write. Its preparation would have been impossible without the help of so many people, some of whom we are bound to forget to thank. So if that person happens to be you, please forgive us. Of course, our main thanks must go to the many authors who have willingly given of their time to bring this project to completion. Without you, this text would have been impossible.

Butterworth Heinemann have been remarkably patient, though we have tested their abilities to an extreme. They have an enviable knack of persuading orthopaedic surgeons like ourselves to keep to time, without causing offence. But in support, and without whom no editing whatsoever would have occurred, particularly special thanks go to Jenny, Linda, Hazel, Pam, Maureen, Sophie, Martina and Suesan. You are all wonderful, the lot of you.

# 1

# The revision problem

Allan E. Gross

More than 800 000 total hip replacements are done world-wide each year[1]. Revision arthroplasty of the hip comprised 17% of all hip replacements with a range of 14–28% in 1991–1992 in the USA[2]. The incidence of revision arthroplasty of the hip increased by 18% in 1992 in the USA compared to 9% for primary hip replacement[3] and will in all probability continue to rise. Revision arthroplasty of the hip is now a problem facing all orthopaedic surgeons who do hip replacement surgery not just those working in tertiary care centres. It is also obvious that complex revisions will have to be performed in tertiary care centres by surgeons with special expertise and resources. The economics of revision hip surgery makes this procedure very unpopular for hospitals and surgeons[3,4]; however, the profession must be held responsible for repairing problems that at least to some degree are iatrogenic.

This book has been written to provide information for orthopaedic surgeons who perform routine hip surgery and for those who wish to accept the more challenging complex cases.

The goals for revision arthroplasty are to relieve pain and improve function for the patient. This can be accomplished by insertion of a new implant with a stable interface and restoration or at least near restoration of the anatomy.

Achieving a stable interface may be done with cemented[5,6] or uncemented components[7,8]. Osteolysis caused by wear debris, abrasion or inflammation may make this task extremely difficult[9–17]. If the failed joint has been infected then the surgeon must decide on a one- or two-stage reconstruction[18,19].

Restoration of the anatomy may be accom-plished by just simply inserting a new implant if there is no loss of bone stock. If there is loss of bone stock on either the pelvic or femoral sides, the deficit must be defined as either contained or uncontained, and dealt with accordingly.

Contained or cavitary defects are more easily dealt with than uncontained defects because by definition there is a weakened but intact skeleton. A contained defect of the acetabulum implies that the columns are intact and the defects are cavitary. On the femoral side a contained defect implies that the cortex of the femur although thinned and even ballooned out is intact. A pelvis or femur with a contained defect can support an implant with a little help. This help can be biological or by implant modification. On the acetabular side impaction grafting with morsellized bone is a biological alternative[19]. Large or asymmetric cups that are designed to make contact with host bone without bone grafting are examples of an implant that may be used where there is a cavitary defect[20].

On the femoral side a contained or cavitary defect can be managed biologically or by implant modification.

The biological solution is impaction bone grafting with a cemented[21,22] or an uncemented implant[23]. Distal fixation with extensively porous coated femoral components and no bone grafting is an alternative[7].

Uncontained or segmental defects are more of a challenge. Small or even moderate defects can be dealt with by placing the implant against host bone without grafting with an acceptable compromise to the anatomy. On the pelvic side a high hip centre allows placement of an uncemented cup against host bone[24,25,26]. On the femoral side a calcar-replacing implant can be utilized[27].

If there is a large segmental pelvic defect with no possibility of placing the implant against host bone then a structural bone graft must be used in order to seat a new cup. If successful, this technique restores bone stock and leg lengths and makes future revision surgery possible. This type of reconstruction has a guarded prognosis, is controversial and should be performed in tertiary care centres[28,29].

A large segmental defect on the femoral side cannot be dealt with by a calcar-replacing prosthesis if it is longer than 3 cm. A structural femoral allograft or a custom prosthesis must be used. Both these techniques have reported good success without as much controversy as on the acetabular side[30,31].

The resource issues of revision arthroplasty of the hip are significant. It is the responsibility of the orthopaedic surgeon who accepts these cases to have a variety of implants and banked bone accessible. He or she must be well versed in a comprehensive surgical exposure that allows access to the anterior and posterior aspects of the pelvis and femur. He or she must be aware of and be able to treat the higher incidence of complications that occur in revision surgery[32]. Finally, there are some failed hip implants that are not amenable to any kind of reconstruction and must be treated by fusion[33] or excision arthroplasty[34,35].

The purpose of this text is to describe the various techniques and results for revision arthroplasty of the hip. In the early years of total hip replacement revisions were carried out for infection and implant failure. As surgical techniques and biomaterials improved the joints lasted longer so that loosening and bone lysis became the most common reasons for revision. The technology of both cemented and uncemented hip replacement has continued to improve with the result that younger and more active patients are undergoing this operation. Component wear with and without loosening is becoming increasingly more important as a failure mechanism in this high demand patient because of the associated bone lysis[36,37].

Loss of bone stock due to loosening and abrasion, stress shielding or osteolysis is the major problem in revision arthroplasty of the hip today. Loss of bone stock is detrimental for both cemented and cementless techniques. The surgical techniques described in this text all have to address this problem and do so by different means. No single technique is the answer for all revisions with different magnitudes of bone loss, and different patient profiles. It is hoped that the reader will be able to understand the principles and develop a more comprehensive approach to this difficult surgical problem.

## References

1. Herberts, P.G., Stromberg, C.N. and Malchau, H. (1995) Revision hip surgery. The challenge. In *Total Hip Revision Surgery* (J.O. Galante, A.G. Rosenberg and J.J. Callaghan, eds) Bristol-Myers Squibb/Zimmer Orthopaedic Symposium Series, New York: Raven Press, pp. 1–15.
2. Keller, R.B. (1995) Outcomes research in revision hip arthroplasty. In *Total Hip Revision Surgery* (J.O. Galante, A.G. Rosenberg and J.J. Callaghan, eds) Bristol-Myers Squibb/Zimmer Orthopaedic Symposium Series, New York: Raven Press, pp. 215–220.
3. Healy, W.L. (1995) The cost of primary and revision total hip arthroplasty. In *Total Hip Revision Surgery* (J.O. Galante, A.G. Rosenberg and J.J. Callaghan, eds) Bristol-Myers Squibb/Zimmer Orthopaedic Symposium Series, New York: Raven Press, pp. 231–236.
4. Bass, G.B. (1995) Hip revision surgery. A hospital administrators perspective. In *Total Hip Revision Surgery* (J.O. Galante, A.G. Rosenberg and J.J. Callaghan, eds) Bristol-Myers Squibb/Zimmer Orthopaedic Symposium Series, New York: Raven Press, pp. 237–241.
5. Estok, D.M. and Harris, W.H. (1994) Long term results of cemented femoral revision using second generation techniques. An average 11 year follow-up evaluation. *Clin. Orthop.*, **299**, 190–203.
6. Stromberg, C.W., Herberts, P.G. and Hultmark, P.N. (1995) Cemented acetabular revisions. In *Total Hip Revision Surgery* (J.O. Galante, A.G. Rosenberg and J.J.Callaghan, eds) Bristol-Myers Squibb/Zimmer Orthopaedic Symposium Series, New York: Raven Press, pp. 311–316.
7. Engh, C.A. and Macalino, G.E. (1995) Clinical results of cementless revision surgery. Are we doing better using extensively coated stems? In *Total Hip Revision Surgery* (J.O. Galante, A.G. Rosenberg and J.J. Callaghan, eds) Bristol-Myers Squibb/Zimmer Orthopaedic Symposium Series, New York: Raven Press, pp. 295–303.
8. Jasty, M. and Harris, W.H. (1995) Cementless acetabular revisions. In *Total Hip Revision Surgery* (J.O. Galante, A.G. Rosenberg and J.J. Callaghan, eds) Bristol-Myers Squibb/Zimmer Orthopaedic Symposium Series, New York: Raven Press, pp. 317–323.
9. Freeman, M.A.R., Bradley, G.W. and Revell, P.A. (1982) Observations upon the interface between bone and polymethylmethacrylate cement. *J. Bone Joint Surg.*, **64B**, 489.
10. Goldring, S.R., Schiller, A.I., Roelke, M.S. et al. (1986) Formation of a synovial-like membrane at the bone cement interface. *Arthritis Rheum.*, **29**, 836.
11. Goldring, S.R., Schiller, A.L., Roelke, M. et al. (1983) The synovial-like membrane at the bone cement interface in loose total hip replacements and its proposed role in bone lysis. *J. Bone Joint Surg.*, **65A**, 575.
12. Goodman, S.B., Schatzker, J., Sumner-Smith, G. et al. (1985) The effect of polymethylmethacrylate on bone: an experimental study. *Arch. Orthop. Trauma Surg.*, **104**, 150.
13. Howie, D., Oakeshott, R., Manthy, B. et al. (1987) Bone resorption in the presence of polyethylene wear particles. *J. Bone Joint Surg.*, **69B**, 165.

14. Jasty, M.J., Floyd, W.E., Schiller, A.L. et al. (1986) Localized osteolysis in stable, non-septic total hip replacement. *J. Bone Joint Surg.*, **68A**, 912.

15. Linder, L., Lindberg, L. and Carlsson, A. (1983) Aseptic loosening of hip prostheses. *Clin. Orthop.*, **175**, 93.

16. Pazzaglia, U.E., Ceciliani, L., Wilkinson, M.J. et al. (1985) Involvement of metal particles in loosening of metal-plastic total hip prostheses. *Arch. Orthop. Trauma Surg.*, **104**, 164.

17. Revell, P.A., Weightman, B., Freeman, M.A.R. et al. (1978) The production and biology of polyethylene wear debris. *Arch. Orthop. Trauma Surg.*, **91**, 167.

18. Buckholz, H.W., Elson, R.A., Engebrocht, B. et al. (1981) Management of deep infection of total hip replacement. *J. Bone Joint Surg.*, **63B**, 353.

19. Sloof, T.J., Schimmel, J.W. and Buma, P. (1993) Cemented fixation with bone grafts: orthopaedic clinics of North America. *Controversies in Total Hip Replacement*, **24**, No. 4, 667–677.

20. Tanzer, M., Drucker, D., Jasty, M. et al. (1992) Revision of acetabular components with an uncemented Harris–Galante porous-coated prosthesis. *J. Bone Joint Surg.*, **74A**, 987–994.

21. Gie, G.A., Linder, L., Ling, R.S.M. et al. (1993) Contained morsellized allograft in revision total hip arthroplasty: surgical techniques. *Orthop. Clin. North Am.*, **24**, 4, 717–727.

22. Gie, G.E., Linder, L. and Ling, R.S.M. (1993) Impacted cancellous allografts and cement for revision total hip arthroplasty. *J. Bone Joint Surg.*, **75B**, 1, 14–21.

23. Gustilo, R.D. and Pasternak, H.S. (1988) Revision total hip arthroplasty with a titanium in growth prosthesis and bone grafting for failed cemented femoral component loosening. *Clin. Orthop.*, **235**, 111–119.

24. Kwong, L.M., Jasty, M. and Harris, W.H. (1993) High failure rate of bulk femoral head allografts in total hip acetabular reconstructions at 10 years. *J. Arthroplasty*, **8**, 341–346.

25. Russotti, G.M. and Harris, W.H. (1991) Proximal placement of the acetabular component in total hip replacement. A long term follow-up study. *J. Bone Joint Surg.*, **73A**, 587–592.

26. Schutzer, S.F. and Harris, W.H. (1994) High placement of porous coated acetabular components in complex total hip arthroplasty. *J. Arthroplasty*, **9**, 359–367.

27. Head, W.C., Wagner, R.A., Emerson, R.H. and Malinin, T.I. (1993) Restoration of femoral bone stock in revision total hip arthroplasty. *Orthop. Clin. North Am.* **24**, No. 4, 697–703.

28. Gross, A.E. (1995) Reconstruction of the acetabulum. In *Total Hip Revision Surgery* (J.O. Galante, A.G.Rosenberg and J.J. Callaghan, eds) Bristol-Myers Squibb/Zimmer Orthopaedic Symposium Series, New York: Raven Press, pp. 335–345.

29. Brick, G.W., Tsahakis, P.J., Sledge, C.B. (1995) Solid allograft reconstruction of acetabular deficiencies. In *Total Hip Revision Surgery* (J.O. Galante, A.G. Rosenberg and J.J. Callaghan, eds) Bristol-Myers Squibb/Zimmer Orthopaedic Symposium Series, New York: Raven Press, pp. 325–333.

30. Allan, D.G., Lavoie, G.J., McDonald, S. et al. (1991) Proximal femoral allografts in revision hip arthroplasty. *J. Bone Joint Surg.*, **73B**, 235–238.

31. Malkani, A.L., Sim, F.H. and Chao, E.Y.S. (1993) Custom-made segmental femoral replacement prosthesis in revision total hip arthroplasty. *Orthop. Clin. North Am.*, **24**, No. 4, 727–733.

32. Allan, D.G., Lavoie, G. and Gross, A.E. (1991) Complications of small fragment allograft reconstruction in revision total hip arthroplasty. In *Complications of Limb Salvage 6th International Symposium, Montreal* (Ken Brown ed.) Published by ISOLS, pp. 285–287.

33. Kostuik, J. and Alexander, D. (1984). Arthrodesis for failed arthroplasty of the hip. *Clin. Orthop.* **188**, 173–182.

34. Harris, W.H. and White, R.E. Jr (1982) Resection arthroplasty for non-septic failure of total hip arthroplasty. *Clin. Orthop.*, **171**, 62.

35. Grauer, J.D., Amstutz, H.C., O'Carroll, F. et al. (1989) Resection arthroplasty of the hip. *J. Bone Joint Surg.*, **71A**, 669–678.

36. Maloney, W.J., Jasty, M., Rosenberg, A. et al. (1990) Bone lysis in well fixed cemented femoral components. *J. Bone Joint Surg.*, **72B**, 966–970.

37. Maloney, W.J., Jasty, M., Harris, W.H. et al. (1990) Endosteal erosion in association with stable uncemented femoral components. *J. Bone Joint Surg.*, **72A**, 1025–1034.

# 2

# Particle disease

Donald W. Howie

Excessive wear particle accumulation may contribute to periprosthetic bone loss and prosthesis loosening. A critical analysis of current and new designs of hip prostheses should, therefore, include an assessment of the potential for a prosthesis to generate excessive wear debris. To do this one needs to be aware of the history of excessive bone loss in relation to potential sources of wear debris, to understand the movement of periprosthetic fluid and migration of wear particles, and to appreciate the effects of particles on cells and how these may relate to cellular mechanisms of bone resorption.

## Periprosthetic osteolysis

A major concern in joint replacement surgery is periprosthetic bone loss. Our research has explored

the hypothesis, based on the work of Willert and Semlitch[1] and Vernon-Roberts and Freeman[2], that wear particles induce a cellular response which causes bone resorption and loosening. The emphasis in our research has previously been the relationship between wear particles produced at the articulating interfaces and loosening. It is now appreciated that wear particles from all interfaces may cause the particular type of bone loss associated with wear particles, termed periprosthetic osteolysis.

The histological section in Figure 2.1 shows the absence of osteolysis beneath a Smith–Peterson cup after many years implantation. There are changes in the bone distribution due to remodelling and loosening but there is not the irregular bone loss that we have come to associate with wear particle induced osteolysis.

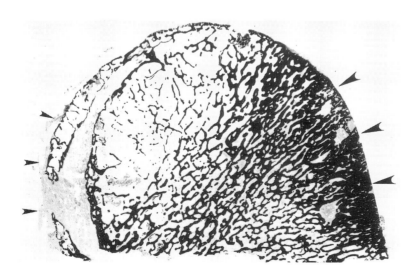

**Figure 2.1** An undecalcified coronal section of a femoral head beneath a cementless Smith–Peterson metal resurfacing hemi-arthroplasty seven years following insertion. The calcified bone is stained black by the Von Kossa technique. The superior weight-bearing area (large arrows) is eburnated and trabecular thickening is evident. On the inferior non-weight-bearing surface (small arrows) mature connective tissue is seen. Few metal particles or macrophages were seen in this tissue (haematoxylin and eosin, Von Kossa stain).

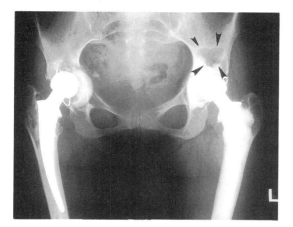

**Figure 2.2** Radiograph of bilateral total hip replacements. The left ilium has an area of severe osteolysis (arrows).

The radiograph in Figure 2.2 at medium term review shows bilateral total hip replacements. The left ilium has the type of severe bone loss that we attribute to excessive wear particle production. Why has this occurred so quickly and to such an extent?

An important concept in understanding the variability in the amount of osteolysis is that this type of periprosthetic bone loss may occur throughout the duration of prosthesis implantation. If wear from the articulating surfaces is excessive, bone loss will occur prior to obvious loosening. Also wear particles may be generated by fretting due to micromovement at interfaces prior to loosening being detectable to naked eye inspection[3]. If slight loosening occurs, which is asymptomatic, then small amounts of movement may cause production of large amounts of wear debris and some bone loss may occur. The result is that after a number of years' implantation, but prior to the patient's symptoms necessitating revision, the amount of bone loss may range from radiographically undetectable to severe.

## Origin of wear particles

What, then, are the potential sources of excessive wear particle production? These may be classified into those from the prosthesis–bone interface and those from the prosthesis–prosthesis interface, which may have been designed to be articulating or non-articulating.

## Prosthesis–bone interface

The prosthesis–bone interface is a potential source of wear and any material moving against bone will produce wear debris. Obviously some designs move more than others while some materials are more wear resistant than others.

### Metal–bone interface

The metal–bone interface is a potential source of debris, be it from press-fit metal stems which often show shiny areas on the stems due to burnishing or from the metal heads of hemiarthroplasties wearing against bone. Yet the amount of wear in these cases is usually acceptable unless, of course, this debris migrates to another interface, such as to a total hip polyethylene–metal articulation, where three-body wear will occur.

Incompletely porous coated stems, despite being ingrown proximally, may show burnishing of their distal surfaces indicating release of wear particles from where their non-coated surfaces abrade against bone. These particles and larger fragments and beads also may migrate to other interfaces.

### Polymer–bone interface

The cement–bone interface is a potent source of wear particles, as evidenced by the smooth appearance of retrieved femoral and acetabular cement mantles which have abraded on bone (Figure 2.3).

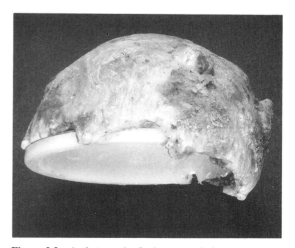

**Figure 2.3** A photograph of a loose acetabular component with polishing of the cement due to abrasion against bone and resultant release of cement debris.

Other implant designs having polymer–bone interfaces have usually resulted in severe wear of the polymer. Examples include uncemented polyethylene cups which have been associated with severe osteolysis. Isoelastic stems are another example.

### Hydroxyapatite–bone interface

Hydroxyapatite coating of implants is appealing. We have previously observed hydroxyapatite fragments separate from the coating of polyethylene acetabular components.

Hydroxyapatite has the potential to degrade and delaminate and for particles to migrate to the polyethylene articulation, where they have recently been reported to cause excessive wear and osteolysis[4].

## Prosthesis–prosthesis articulation

### Metal–metal articulation

Prosthesis–prosthesis articulations are a potential source of large numbers of wear particles which are released into the surrounding tissues. Inappropriately designed metal–metal articulations of cobalt–chrome alloy may result in moderate wear and the accumulation of metal wear particles in the tissues. This has been associated with bone destruction and histological examination of the grey stained tissue reveals fibrous tissues, a macrophage infiltrate in association with metal wear particles, necrosis and osteoclastic resorption of bone. Occasional lymphocytes and lymphocytic aggregates are seen.

Some of our long-term retrievals of McKee prostheses after approximately twenty years' service have shown a surprisingly benign tissue appearance and very few wear particles. Hence the renewed interest in these bearings.

### Metal–polyethylene articulation

Prostheses with metal–polyethylene articulations have served well but remain susceptible to wear, and severe lysis is not uncommonly seen on long-term radiographs. Histological examination of the tissues around metal-on-polyethylene arthroplasties demonstrate a common pattern; the tissues are infiltrated with varying numbers of macrophages and multinucleate giant cells are common while lymphocytic aggregates are only occasionally present (Figures 2.4, 2.5). The tissues usually contain large numbers of highly birefringent polyethylene particles and variable numbers of metal particles.

### Three-body wear

Three-body wear occurs due to interposition of a material harder than one of the articulating surfaces and remains a problem with polyethylene articulations due commonly to cement particle interposition (Figure 2.6). The release of metal particles, wire and beads from non-cemented prostheses are also capable of causing this severe three-body wear (Figure 2.7). This type of wear results in scratching of the metal articulating surface and if a titanium articulating surface is used the problem is compounded.

Aluminium oxide ceramic articulating against itself has been reported to be more resistant to wear in ideal conditions, but disastrous wear may occur.

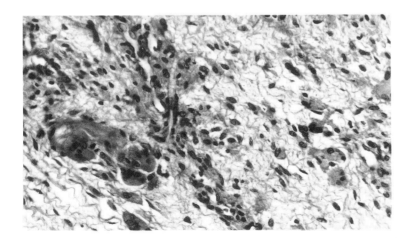

**Figure 2.4** Photomicrograph of the acetabular connective tissue at the bone–cement interface of a slightly loose cemented metal-on-polyethylene arthroplasty. It shows a group of macrophages and occasional multinucleated giant cells in a collagenous matrix (haematoxylin and eosin, x400).

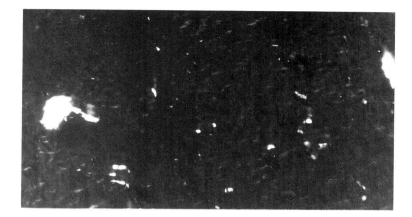

Figure 2.5 Photomicrograph of the same section shown in Figure 2.4 viewed by polarized light. It shows small highly birefringent particles in macrophages, and large particles in multinucleated giant cells (haematoxylin and eosin, x400).

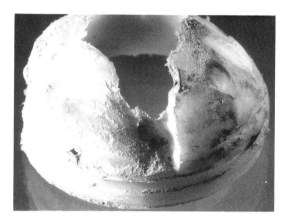

Figure 2.6 Photograph of a polyethylene Muller acetabular component retrieved eight years following insertion. There has been complete penetration of the component which had become loose in the cement mantle. Large cement particles were seen on the articulating surface of the component and these probably produced three-body wear.

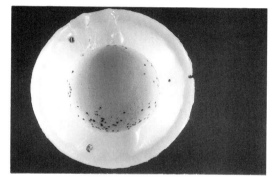

Figure 2.7 Photograph of a polyethylene acetabular liner from a porous coated total hip replacement. The beads from the porous coating have migrated to the acetabular articulating surface and become embedded in the polyethylene. They are an important cause of three-body wear.

## Prosthesis–prosthesis non-articulating interfaces

### Prosthesis–cement interface

In the past we have assumed that no movement occurred at modular interfaces, or what little that did was unimportant. This has changed. An example is the prosthesis–cement interface. It is becoming increasingly clear that movement between stem and cement may produce large amounts of metal and cement debris. Cemented stems may be slightly loose and yet function well for many years, during which large numbers of wear particles may be produced. This is confirmed by examination of cemented stems which show evidence of abrasion which generates metal and cement debris.

Titanium stems may be particularly prone to wear and clinical reports of wear and loosening support this as a cause of loosening[5]. We retrieved a titanium alloy stem which was particularly interesting in that the stem remained firmly fixed in the cement distally yet, after sectioning the stem, we found abrasion of the proximo-anterior surface with polishing of the cement and metal in this region. It may be that titanium alloy stems deform to the extent that wear occurs before discernible loosening.

Thus the stem–cement interface is a source of wear and release of metal and cement debris. Polished stems, which we have occasionally retrieved after long-term successful function, have been associated with little osteolysis. This, and the observations of Ling and co-workers[3], support

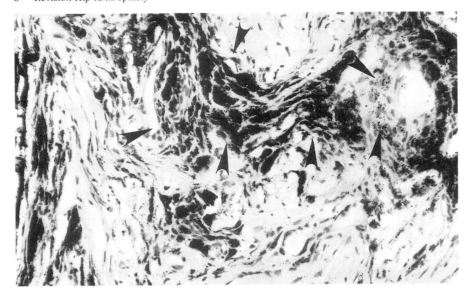

**Figure 2.8** A photomicrograph of the black stained acetabular connective tissue around a loose titanium plasma sprayed backing to a loose acetabular component. It shows large numbers of metal particles within macrophages and extracellularity (arrows). There was severe bone resorption (haematoxylin and eosin, x100).

the concept that polished stems may minimize wear. Of particular interest are their observations of the appearance of retrieved matt stems on which they described a regular pattern of burnishing despite the stems being macroscopically solid. They concluded that fretting was occurring at apparently solid stem–cement interfaces and that if matt stems were used then excessive wear debris would be produced.

Severe wear may also occur on the surface of those acetabular components which did not remain adequately fixed in cement (Figure 2.8).

### Modular prostheses

Wear particles may also be generated from movement at any of the interfaces of a modular prosthesis, as observed on inadequately designed head neck tapers, potentially at modular stem junctions, and at screw-cup junctions.

### Particle migration and prosthesis loosening

Given that there are various potential sources of wear debris, how then do wear particles migrate to reach bone or have an effect on bone. It is important to understand that the tissue response to an implant is to attempt to isolate the implant, thus forming a relatively enclosed system in which joint fluid may circulate, but which can still affect and

be affected by the surrounding tissues. This fluid has the potential to move to and fro along interfaces so that wear occurring at one interface will affect other interfaces as well as the surrounding tissues. Fortunately there are mechanisms for clearance of wear products from the joint but if wear particle production is excessive then an adverse tissue response will occur.

To study the relationship between particle migration and the degree of loosening we used a loosening grading system and examined numerous femoral heads beneath double cup resurfacing arthroplasties[6].

Histological examination demonstrated the presence of small polyethylene particles in the superior regions of the bone–cement interface of solidly fixed femoral components with stable interfaces. These particles were seen within macrophages in the marrow spaces and in the very thin, incomplete cellular connective tissue separating bone from cement. Since these particles were found in areas a considerable distance from the joint cavity, it is proposed that small polyethylene particles migrate along the interface between solidly fixed components. It may also be possible that macrophages already containing these particles migrate along these interfaces.

We and others have shown by arthrographic studies that joint fluid penetrates the implant–bone interface. Fluid is seen at the proximal bone–cement interface of solid femoral stems, invariably reaches the bone–cement interface of cemented sockets, and may reach part of the implant–bone interface around solidly fixed cementless components. Given that the capsule is a potent producer of cell mediators capable of stimulating bone resorption[7], then the migration of this fluid along the bone–implant interface could well explain the osteolysis seen around solid uncemented stems.

We have seen localized radiolucent areas containing wear particles in resurfaced femoral heads and necks and similar resorption is increasingly being reported around uncemented acetabular components, evidence suggesting that fluid may migrate into cancellous bone.

Another interesting observation we had made many years ago was the presence of small areas of radiolucency near the tips of apparently solidly fixed stems which at revision had some wear of the acetabular component. Histological examination of the tissue at the site of the distal lucencies showed a macrophage infiltrate and the presence of small polyethylene particles.

We were unable to explain this fully until the work of Anthony et al.[8] who have proposed that joint fluid containing wear particles may move along the space between the stem and its surrounding cement mantle and exit through defects in the latter to reach the periprosthetic bone. The presence of mediators of resorption or pressure effects cause the scalloped appearance of bone resorption at a distance from the joint. Clearly wear particles may migrate to a number of sites as summarized in Table 2.1.

**Table 2.1   The sites to which particulate debris may migrate**

| |
| --- |
| Intra-articular |
| Prosthesis–bone interface |
|   cement–bone |
|   metal–bone |
|   polymer–bone |
|   other–bone |
| Prosthesis–cement interface |
| Intra–osseous |
| Extra–osseous |
|   regional |
|   systematic |

## The effect of wear particles on cells and tissues

Having summarized the potential sources of wear particles and how they may migrate with joint fluid I now wish to briefly address the tissue and cellu-

lar response to wear debris. We have studied this by *in vitro* and *in vivo* experiments which we have attempted to correlate with human observations. We have undertaken a number of studies involving intra-articular injection of wear particles into rat knees.

A summary of these findings is that injection of cobalt–chrome particles into rat knee joints causes an acute inflammatory response followed by a macrophage infiltrate, necrosis and a lymphocyte response (Figure 2.9). Electron microscopy shows that this is followed by proliferation of macrophages and synoviocytes which have increased secretory activity. Long-term studies show the necrosis and macrophage response persist as does the presence of particles, although some are cleared from the joint[9]. There were differences in response between different materials as shown by the lack of necrosis and a smaller initial macrophage response to aluminium oxide particles[10].

Also we prepared polyethylene particles in a wear simulator. Injection of these particles produces the typical appearance seen around prostheses with a polyethylene articulating surface. Large shards of polyethylene and also aggregates of small particles were contained within multinucleated giant cells. Particles less than 5 µm caused a mononuclear cell response[11].

A rat model was developed in which repeated injections were undertaken of polyethylene wear particles injected into a rat knee in which acrylic plugs had previously been inserted into the distal femur[12]. Polyethylene particles were found at the

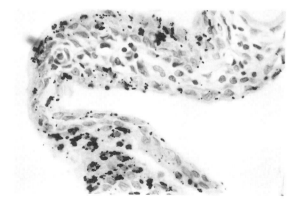

**Figure 2.9**  Photomicrograph of rat knee synovial tissue laden with metallic particles in association with macrophages after a three-week course of twice-weekly intra-articular injections of cobalt–chrome particles of less than three micrometres in diameter (haematoxylin & eosin, x600).

## Cross section of femur

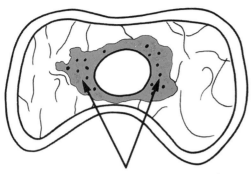

## particles and bone resorption

**Figure 2.10**   Diagram to represent a transverse section of the distal rat femur. It shows particle accumulation and replacement of bone by connective tissue after injection of particles into the joint adjacent to an intramedullary cement plug.

interface between the cement plug and bone (Figure 2.10). The variability of the response, however, suggested that micromovement or synovial infiltration are necessary to allow particles to easily access the interface. This model supports our hypothesis that in the absence of either infection, loading or macromovement at the interface, one sees a response to prosthesis wear particles which have migrated to the prosthesis–bone interface.

## Cell mediators of bone resorption

The problem with the *in vivo* studies described above is the difficulty in making quantitative comparisons and isolating cell mechanisms and we have therefore used *in vitro* studies to compare the effects on cells of different particles and to relate this to mechanisms of bone resorption.

We know that the periprosthetic fluid produced by the capsular tissue contains inflammatory mediators and macrophages are known to be producers of a large number of these potent mediators[13,14]. These mediators, prostaglandin $E_2$ ($PGE_2$), interleukin 1 (IL-1), tumour necrosis factor (TNF) and interleukin 6 (IL-6), have been implicated in the stimulation of bone resorption. An hypothesis to explain bone loss is that when macrophages phagocytose wear particles they release mediators which either directly, or via indirect mechanisms possibly

involving the osteoblast, stimulate osteoclastic bone resorption.

We have developed standard methods for characterization of size, size distribution and shape of particles, and therefore have been able to compare the effects of similar numbers of particles of different materials[15].

We and others had previously concentrated on the toxic effects of particles which might cause an initial release of inflammatory mediators, followed by cell death and fibrosis. It might be, however, that stimulatory effects of less toxic materials are more deleterious due to continuing production of inflammatory mediators. To test this hypothesis we compared the effects of particles of a material having known toxic effects — cobalt–chrome — to a supposedly more biocompatible less toxic material, titanium alloy.

Rat macrophages were exposed to varying concentrations of these particles and the degree of cell toxicity and the level of inflammatory mediators in the supernatant was measured. Titanium alloy was less toxic compared to cobalt–chrome, as expected, but titanium alloy caused increased inflammatory mediator release, which it could be argued is more important in causing bone resorption[16].

To examine the response to polymers we initially used latex beads and found that there was little response at medium concentrations of particles but compared to metals high concentrations later caused mediator release, and others have demonstrated this release[17]. We have recently been able to prepare small polyethylene particles of approximately 1 µm diameter and preliminary studies show polyethylene particles cause variable release of mediators[18]. It may be that the response to these polymer particles is due to a non-specific response to phagocytosis and the continuing presence in a cell.

We have begun further studies of the role of these inflammatory mediators in the osteoclast–osteoblast relationship and how they may cause bone resorption. The aim of these studies is to define the potential pathways for osteoclast stimulation and early results suggest a mechanism involving the osteoblast[19].

All these studies are *in vitro* and should not be directly transposed to the human situation, but help to define mechanisms that may occur in humans.

## Summary

In summary, bone resorption is probably induced by inflammatory mediators. These mediators are released in response to wear debris of all materials. Our research suggests, however, that there may be differences in the amount of released mediators in response to different materials. Synovial fluid movement allows communication between the different prosthetic interfaces and the periprosthetic tissues, and this explains a number of the features of wear particle disease.

Importantly it should be remembered that there are other mechanisms for bone loss including mechanical effects, remodelling and possibly the effects of movement and hydrostatic effects as well as infection.

In conclusion it is suggested that when assessing the value of a current or proposed hip prosthesis, one should apply the following criteria. Is movement possible at any of the interfaces of this prosthesis and, if so, are the materials and design features appropriate to prevent excessive wear? If not, then wear particle induced bone resorption will eventually occur.

## Acknowledgements

This work was undertaken in association with the staff of the following Departments and the author acknowledges their assistance: Department of Orthopaedic Surgery and Trauma, Royal Adelaide Hospital; Department of Pathology and Department of Orthopaedics and Trauma, University of Adelaide; Division of Tissue Pathology, and Medical Illustration and Electron Microscopy Units of the Institute of Medical and Veterinary Science. The author acknowledges the assistance of Professor B. Vernon-Roberts, Dr R. Garrett, Mr D. Haynes, Ms M. McGee, Mrs J. McLean, Ms S. Hay, Ms S. Rogers, Dr M. Pearcy, and Mrs E. Patterson.

## Research support

This research was supported in part by grants from the Dawes Research Fellowship and Royal Adelaide Hospital Research Foundation, the Adelaide Bone and Joint Research Foundation, Australian Orthopaedic Association and Royal Australasian College of Surgeons, and National Health and Medical Research Council.

## References

1. Willert, H.G. and Semlitsch, M. (1977) Reactions of the articular capsule to wear products of artificial joint prostheses. *J. Biomed. Mater. Res.*, **11**, 157–164.
2. Vernon-Roberts, B. and Freeman, M.A.R. (1977) The tissue response to total joint replacement prostheses. In *The Scientific Basis of Joint Replacement* (S.A.U. Swanson and M.A.R. Freeman, eds) Tunbridge Wells, Kent: Pitman Medical Publishing, p. 86.
3. Hale, D.G., Lee, A.J.C., Ling, R.S.M. and Hooper, R.M. (1991) Debris production by the femoral component in the cemented total hip arthroplasty. *J. Bone Joint Surg.*, **73B**(Suppl I) 18.
4. Bloebaum, R.D. and Dupont, J.A. (1993) Osteolysis from a press-fit hydroxyapatite-coated implant. A case study. *J. Arthroplasty*, **8**(2), 195–202.
5. Witt, J.D. and Swann, M. (1991) Metal wear and tissue response in failed titanium alloy total hip replacements. *J. Bone Joint Surg.*, **73B**, 559–563.
6. Howie, D.W., Cornish, B.L. and Vernon-Roberts, B. (1990) Resurfacing hip arthroplasty: classification of loosening and the role of prosthesis wear particles. *Clin. Orthop.* **255**, 144–159.
7. Ohlin, A. (1989) Socket wear, loosening and bone resorption after total hip arthroplasty. Doctoral Dissertation, Lund University.
8. Anthony, P.P., Gie, G.A., Howie, C.R. and Ling, R.S.M. (1990) Localised endosteal bone lysis in relation to the femoral components of cemented total hip arthroplasties. *J. Bone Joint Surg.*, **72B**, 971–979.
9. Howie, D.W. and Vernon-Roberts, B. (1988) Long-term effects of intraarticular cobalt–chrome alloy wear particles in rats. *J. Arthroplasty*, **3**(4), 327–336.
10. Howie, D.W. and Vernon-Roberts, B. (1988) The synovial macrophage response to aluminium oxide ceramic and cobalt–chrome alloy wear particles in rats. *Biomaterials*, **9**, 442–48.
11. Howie, D.W., Manthey, B., Hay, S. and Vernon-Roberts, B. (1993) The synovial response to intraarticular injections of polyethylene wear particles. *Clin. Orthop.*, **292**, 352–357.
12. Howie, D.W., Vernon-Roberts, B., Oakeshott, R. and Manthey, B. (1988) A rat model of resorption of bone at the cement–bone interface in the presence of polyethylene wear particles. *J. Bone Joint. Surg.*, **70A**, 257.
13. Goldring, S.R., Jasty, M., Roelke, M.S. et al. (1986) Formation of a synovial-like membrane at the bone–cement interface. Its role in bone resorption and implant loosening after total hip replacement. *Arthritis Rheum.*, **29**, 836–42.
14. Horowitz, S.M., Salvati, E., Glasser, D.B. and Lane, J.M. (1991) Prostaglandin E2 is increased in the synovial fluid of patients with aseptic loosening. *Trans. 37th Ann. Meet. Orthop. Res. Soc.*, **16**(2), 335.
15. Rogers, S.D., Pearcy, M.J., Hay, S.J. et al. (1993) A method for production and characterization of metal prosthesis wear particles. *J. Orthop. Res.* **11**, 856–864.
16. Haynes, D.R., Rogers, S.D., Hay, S. et al. (1993) The differences in toxicity and release of bone-resorbing mediators induced by titanium and cobalt–chrome alloy wear particles. *J. Bone Joint Surg.*, **75A**, 825–834.
17. Murray, D.W. and Rushton, N. (1990) Macrophages stimulate bone resorption when they phagocytose particles. *J. Bone Joint Surg.*, **72B**, 988–992.
18. Howie, D.W., Rogers, S.D., Haynes, D.R. and Pearcy, M.J. (1994) The role of small polyethylene wear particles in inducing the release of mediators known to stimulate bone resorption. *Trans. 40th Ann. Meet., Orthop. Res. Soc.*, New Orleans, U.S.A. February.
19. Ohta, S., Graves, S., Rogers, S.D. et al. (1994) Osteoblasts release IL-6 and PGE2 in response to TiCl3 and conditioned media from macrophages exposed to TiAIV wear particles. *Trans. 40th Ann. Meet. Orthop. Res. Soc.*, **19**, 149.

# 3

# A systematic approach to revision arthroplasty of the hip

Allan E. Gross

The goal of revision arthroplasty of the hip is to achieve a stable implant with restoration of anatomy. This may be achieved relatively easily or with great difficulty depending on the available bone stock.

The primary goal is to implant new components against host knee with restoration of anatomy and leg lengths. This can be done with or without the use of cement depending on the characteristics of the patient and the preferences of the surgeon[1–15].

If the primary goal cannot be achieved, the secondary goal would be to achieve stable components and restore anatomy and leg lengths but with help from bone grafts or prosthetic design. If bone graft is used it is either morsellized or non-circumferential (cortical strut) so that the implant is supported primarily by host bone. Some implants are designed to compensate for minimal to moderate loss of bone stock. Femoral components with calcar-replacing stems and several neck lengths, and oblong asymmetric cups are examples of this[16,17].

When the bone loss is more severe and the implants cannot be stabilized primarily against host bone, then a decision has to be made whether to sacrifice or to restore anatomy and leg lengths. If the components can be stabilized primarily against host bone with acceptable sacrifice of anatomy, then the tertiary goal is achieved. The high hip centre is an example of this[16]. If the loss of bone stock is very severe and the components cannot be stabilized primarily against host bone then structural grafts or custom implants must be used to restore anatomy and leg lengths. This is the quaternary goal[18–26]. We have used this approach to produce the following classification of revisions:

## Type I

Uncemented or cemented components placed in host bone with restoration of anatomy and leg lengths (Figure 3.1).

## Type II

Uncemented or cemented components supported primarily by host bone but with some minor support by bone graft (i.e. morsellized bone, cortical strut) or by prosthetic design (i.e. calcar-replacing prosthesis, oblong cup), with restoration of anatomy and leg lengths (Figure 3.2).

## Type III

Uncemented or cemented components supported primarily by host bone with acceptable loss of anatomy and leg length (high hip centre) (Figure 3.3).

## Type IV

Uncemented or cemented components supported by structural grafts or custom prostheses with restoration of anatomy and leg lengths (Figures 3.4 and 3.5).

Several factors must be considered before deciding on the type of revision and what type of components to use.

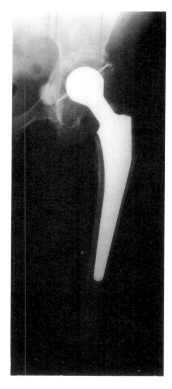

(a)

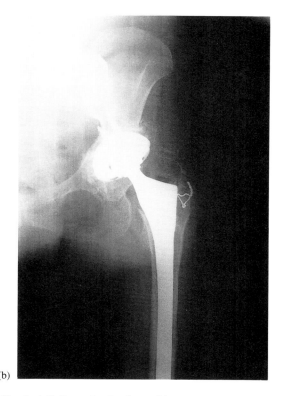

(b)

**Figure 3.1**   Type 1 Revision: a, A.P. X-ray left hip of a 60-year-old female with a loose cemented total hip prosthesis but no significant loss of bone stock on the pelvic or femoral sides. b, A.P. X-ray shortly after revision to an uncemented total hip prosthesis. Bone graft was not necessary on either the pelvic or femoral sides.

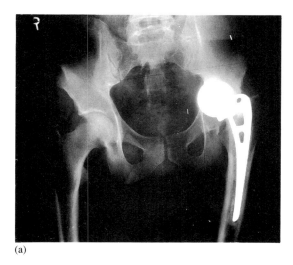

(a)

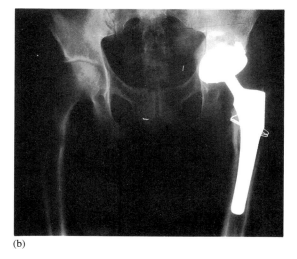

(b)

**Figure 3.2**   Type II Revision: a, A.P. X-ray 9 years after a Moore arthroplasty had been performed for osteonecrosis of the femoral head due to steroids in a 30-year-old male. There is a contained or cavitary loss of bone stock on the pelvic side due to a superomedial protrusion. b, A.P. X-ray 7 years after revision using morcellized allograft bone and a fixed uncemented cup.

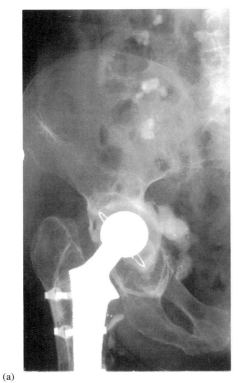

(a)

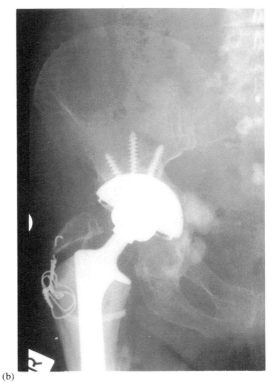

(b)

**Figure 3.3**  Type III Revision: a, A.P. X-ray of a loose cemented right acetabular prosthesis with a severe supero-medial protrusion in a 65-year-old female. b, A.P. X-ray of right hip 3 years after reconstruction with morcellized allograft bone and an uncemented cup placed in a proximal position (high hip centre).

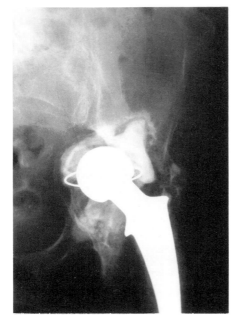

(a)

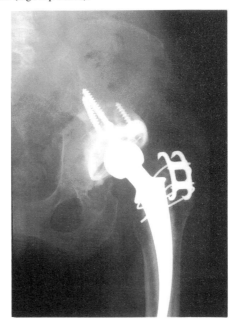

(b)

**Figure 3.4**  Type IV Revision structural acetabular graft: a, A.P. X-ray of left hip in a 65-year-old female showing a loose cemented acetabular component with marked loss of pelvic bone stock. b, A.P. X-ray after revision using a bulk acetabular allograft fixed with a roof reinforcement ring. The cup is cemented.

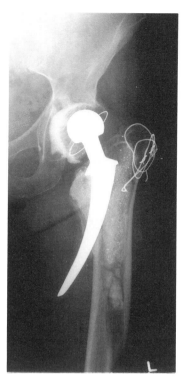

(a)

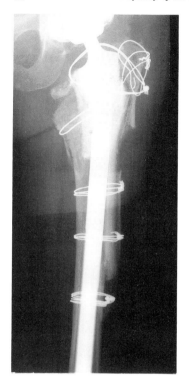

(b)

**Figure 3.5**  Type 4 Revision structural femoral graft: a, A.P. X-ray left hip of a loose cemented perforated femoral component in a 60-year-old female. b, A.P. X-ray left hip 6 months following a structural proximal femoral allograft.

## Patient factors

The level of demand of the patient is determined by age, height, weight, occupation and lifestyle. For example in a high demand patient, restoration of bone stock, and the use of uncemented components would seem more advisable.

In a low demand patient who is unlikely to require another revision, the use of a long-stem cemented component is more acceptable than in a higher demand patient that might require another revision[27].

Loss of bone stock anatomy and leg length discrepancy are crucial factors in decision making. This must be determined accurately prior to surgery. In addition to plain X-rays, Judet views of the pelvis[28] and a CAT scan may be helpful for assessing bone stock.

Infection must be ruled out if suspected. Bone scan, gallium scan, indium scan and hip aspiration may be helpful[29,30,31]. Even if these tests are negative and if at the time of surgery the findings on gross examination or on Gram stain or frozen section are suspicious of infection then in the opinion of the author the reconstruction should be done in two stages if structural grafts are necessary.

## Surgeon factors

Surgeon factors play an important role in decision making about the type of revision and the components to be used. Some surgeons prefer to do all their revisions cementless[7,9] while others use cement[8,11,12]. Some surgeons will not use bone grafts of any type while others will use morsellized graft but not structural. Surgeons who will not use structural grafts either use custom prostheses[33] or are willing to sacrifice some anatomy and leg length to place their components against host bone[34]. In some centres, excision arthroplasty[35,36] or fusion[37] is more accepted by surgeons and patients than in others.

## References

1. Gustilo, R.D. and Pasternak, H.S. (1988) Revision total hip arthroplasty with a titanium ingrowth prosthesis and bone grafting for failed cemented femoral component loosening. *Clin. Orthop.* **235**, 111–119.
2. Harris, W.H., Krushell, R.J. and Galante, J.O. (1988) Results of cementless revisions of total hip arthroplasties using the Harris–Galante prosthesis. *Clin. Orthop.* **235**, 120–126.
3. Gross, A.E., Lavoie, M.V., McDermott, A.G.P. et al. (1985) The use of allograft bone in revision of total hip arthroplasty. *Clin. Orthop.* **197**, 115.
4. Amstutz, H.C., Ma, S. and Jinnah, R.H. (1982) Revision of aseptic loose total hip arthroplasties. *Clin. Orthop.* **170**, 21–33.
5. Callaghan, J.J., Salvati, E.A., Pellicci, P.M. et al. 1985 Results of revision for mechanical failure after cemented total hip replacement, 1979 to 1982. A two to five year follow-up. *J. Bone Joint Surg.* **67A**, 1074–1085.
6. Emerson, R.H. Jr, Head, W.C., Berklacich, F.M. et al. (1989) Noncemented acetabular revision arthroplasty using allograft bone. *Clin. Orthop.* **249**, 30–43.
7. Engh, C.A., Glassman, A.H., Griffin, W.L. et al. (1988) Results of cementless revision for failed cemented total hip arthroplasty. *Clin. Orthop.* **235**, 91–110.
8. Fuchs, M.D., Salvati, E.A., Wilson, P.D. Jr et al. (1988) Results of acetabular revisions with newer cement techniques. *Orthop. Clin. North Am.* **19**, 649–655.
9. Hedley, A.K., Gruen, T.A. and Ruoff, D.P. (1988) Revision of failed total hip arthroplasties with uncemented porous-coated anatomic components. *Clin. Orthop.* **235**, 75–90.
10. Hunter, G.A., Welsh, R.P., Cameron, H.U. et al. (1979) The results of revision of total hip arthroplasty. *J. Bone Joint Surg.*, **61B**, 419–421.
11. Kavanagh, B.E., Ilstrup, D.M. and Fitzgerald, R.H. Jr (1985) Revision total hip arthroplasty. *J. Bone Joint Surg.*, **67A**, 517–526.
12. Pellicci, P.M., Wilson, P.D. Jr, Sledge, C.B. et al. (1982) Revision total hip arthroplasty. *Clin. Orthop.* **170**, 34–41.
13. Pellicci, P.M., Wilson, P.D. Jr, Sledge, C.B. et al. (1985) Long-term results of revision total hip replacement. A follow-up report. *J. Bone Joint Surg.*, **67A**, 513–516.
14. Wilson-MacDonald, J., Morscher, E. and Masar, Z. (1990) Cementless uncoated polyethylene acetabular components in total hip replacement. A review of five to 10 year results. *J. Bone Joint Surg.*, **72B**, 423–430.
15. Pierson, J.L. and Harris, W.H. (1994) Cemented revision for femoral osteolysis in cemented arthroplasties. *J. Bone Joint Surg.*, **76B**, 40–44.
16. Russotti, G.M. and Harris, W.H. (1991) Proximal placement of the acetabular component in total hip arthroplasty. A long-term follow-up study. *J. Bone Joint Surg.*, **73A**, 587–592.
17. Bargar, W.M. (1993) Personal Communication.
18. Gross, A.E. (1992) Revision arthroplasty of the hip using allograft bone. In *Allografts in Orthopaedic Practice* (A.A. Czitrom and A.E. Gross, eds ) Williams & Wilkins, Baltimore, pp. 147–173.
19. Chao, E.Y.S. and Ivins, J.C. (1983) The design and application. In *Tumour Prostheses for Bone and Joint Reconstruction*, Thieme-Stratton, New York, p. 335.
20. Chao, E.Y.S. and Sim, F.H. (1992) Composite fixation of salvage prostheses for the hip and the knee. *Clin. Orthop.* **276**, 91.
21. Unwin, P.S., Cobb, J.P. and Walker, P.S. (1993) Distal femoral arthroplasty using custom-made prosthesis; the first 218 cases. *J. Arthroplasty*, **8**, 259–268.
22. Blunn, G.W., Hua, J., Wait, M.E. and Walker, P.S. (1991) Correlation of stress distribution with bony remodelling in retrieved femora with proximal femoral replacement. In *Complications of Limb Salvage: Prevention, Management and Outcome* (K. Brown ed.) ISOLS, Montreal, pp. 445–450.
23. Markel, M.D., Gottsauner-Wolf, F., Rock, M.G. et al. (1991) A mechanical comparison of six methods of proximal femoral replacement. In *Complications of Limb Salvage* (K. Brown ed.) ISOLS, Montreal, pp. 75–80.
24. Zehr, R.J., Heare, T., Enneking, W.F. et al. (1991) Allograft prosthesis composite vs. megaprosthesis in proximal femoral reconstruction. In *Complications of Limb Salvage* (K. Brown ed.) ISOLS, Montreal, pp. 91–103.
25. Unwin, P.S., Cobb, J.P., Walker, P.S., et al. (1991) Loosening in cemented femoral prostheses: a study of 668 tumour cases. In *Complications of Limb Salvage* (K. Brown ed.) ISOLS, Montreal, pp. 133–137.
26. Wipperman, B., Zwipp, H., Sturm, J. et al. (1991) Complications of endoprosthetic proximal femoral replacement. In *Complications of Limb Salvage* (K. Brown ed.) ISOLS, Montreal, pp. 143–146.
27. Rubash, H.E. and Harris, W.H. (1988) Revision of nonseptic loose cemented femoral components using modern cementing techniques. *Arthroplasty*, **3**, 241.
28. Judet, R., Judet, J. and Letournel E. (1964) Fractures of the acetabulum: classification and surgical approaches for open reduction. *J. Bone Joint Surg.*, **46A**, 1615–1646.
29. Barrack, R.L. and Harris, W.H. (1993) The value of aspiration of the hip joint before revision total hip arthroplasty. *J. Bone Joint Surg.*, **75A**, **1**, 66–76.
30. Gristina, A.G. and Kolkin, J. (1983) Current concepts review. Total joint replacement and sepsis. *J. Bone Joint Surg.*, **65A**, 128–134.
31. Johnson, J.A., Christie, M.J., Sandler, M.P. et al. (1988) Detection of occult infection following total joint arthroplasty using sequential technetium-99m HDP bone scintigraphy and indium-111 WBC imaging. *J. Nucl. Med.*, **29**, 1347–1353.
32. Padgett, D.E., Kull, L., Rosenberg, A. et al. (1993) Revision of the acetabular component without cement after total hip arthroplasty. *J. Bone Joint Surg.*, **75A**, 663–673.
33. Bargar, W.L., Murzic, W.J., Taylor, J.K. et al. (1993) Management of bone loss in revision total hip arthroplasty using custom cementless femoral components. *J. Arthroplasty*, **8**, 245–252.
34. Jasty, M. and Harris, W.H. (1990) Salvage total hip reconstruction in patients with major acetabular bone deficiency using structural femoral head allografts. *J. Bone Joint Surg.*, **72B**, 63.
35. Harris, W.H. and White, R.E. Jr (1982) Resection arthroplasty for non-septic failure of total hip arthroplasty. *Clin. Orthop.*, **171**, 62.
36. Grauer, J.D., Amstutz, H.C., O'Carroll, F. et al. (1989) Resection arthroplasty of the hip. *J. Bone Joint Surg.*, **71A**, 669–678.
37. Kostuik, J. and Alexander, D. (1984) Arthrodesis for failed arthroplasty of the hip. *Clin. Orthop.*, **188**, 173–182.

# 4

# Diagnosis and management of infection

Ian Stockley

Sepsis following arthroplasty surgery remains one of the most devastating complications encountered in orthopaedic surgery. Although the infection rate has fallen considerably over the years following introduction of ultra clean air, body exhaust suits and prophylactic antibiotics, actual numbers of new infected cases are significant in view of the large numbers of arthroplasties now performed.

The consequences of deep infection include not only failure of the involved joint but also the need for further surgical episodes. The clinical result is often far from perfect with a prolonged rehabilitation period and its associated morbidity. Economic losses relate not only to the individual but also to the hospital as the costs of surgery and rehabilitation are much greater with a revision compared to a primary procedure.

The fundamental pathogenic mechanism in biomaterial-centred sepsis is microbial colonization of biomaterials and adjacent damaged tissues. Colonization occurs because bacteria have developed a unique and preferential ability to adhere to inanimate substrata. Microbial adhesion involves a chemical bonding of bacterial extracapsular structures to the surface of an implant. Unfortunately, implant-related sepsis is difficult to treat as adherent bacteria behave in a different way to free floating bacteria as demonstrated by decreased susceptibility to antibiotics. These factors render the usage of antibiotics alone ineffective and radical surgical debridement is mandatory.

In addition to adhesion and colonization, bacteria are also able to produce slime layers. The exopolysaccharide slime acts as an ion exchange resin, enhancing nutrition, moderating susceptibility to phagocytosis and altering the organism's response to antibodies. It also functions in later stages of surface adhesion, aggregation and polymicrobial interaction. Shortly after attachment and adhesion, growth and division accelerate if the environment is appropriate, extracellular polysaccharide polymers are produced that provide additional adhesion to surfaces. The aggregated accumulation of polysaccharides, bacteria, bacterial microcolonies of the same or different species, environmental and host products forms the biofilm. This biofilm matrix serves not only as an adhesive mechanism but also appears to be virulence related. It can resist host defence mechanisms and may also impede the effective penetration of antibiotics.

When an implant is inserted into the body, the implant surface is a ready site for competitive bacterial or tissue colonization. Its free energy sites are awaiting to be occupied by the first available passers by, be they bacteria or host cells. If tissue cells arrive first, the space is occupied and so less space is available for bacterial colonization. If bacteria arrive first, once attached they produce polysaccharide polymers and provide a foundation for further growth and colonization.

## Diagnosis

Deep-seated infection is not always clinically obvious. High-grade infection with cellulitis, abscess or sinus formation is easy to diagnose but most infections today are low grade, caused by organisms which are often skin commensals, and can be difficult to identify. Indeed, these organisms until relatively recently were regarded, by some authorities, as being of no significant value. The patient's clinical history may give clues regarding the possibility of failure being due to sepsis. Problems with wound healing, e.g. leakage from the wound with regular dressing changes, erythema, extensive or frequent antibiotic prescriptions, evacuation of haematoma, or a prolonged clinical recovery should prompt suspicion. Often, on close questioning it becomes apparent that these patients have never really been free of pain and as such have not gained the clinical benefit one normally expects following hip arthroplasty. The possibility of infection must always arise when considering reasons for failure particularly with early clinical failure.

Examination may reveal multiple scars, puckered areas, subcutaneous thickening with induration or a dry sinus. Classical signs of infection with cellulitis and a discharging sinus are often absent. The majority of cases present with well-healed surgical scars.

### Plain radiography

Plain films are the most commonly used investigation used to assess hip pain. It is important to ensure that good quality, comparable anteroposterior and lateral radiographs are obtained so that comparisons can be made. Unfortunately the initial postoperative film is often of poor quality thus making comparison difficult. In the early stages of infection ill-defined bone resorption may be seen but often there is no significant change. In the later stages, lucencies at the cement–bone and cement–prosthesis interfaces become apparent, cement may fracture, components subside and periosteal new bone formation is observed, (Figure 4.1). Aseptic loosening and endosteal lysis can look very similar to the septic hip in its advanced state, apart from the absence of periostitis. The clinical history suggests the diagnosis. If extensive radiolucencies are present within a relatively short time since implantation (e.g. five years) then sepsis is the probable diagnosis.

### Scintigraphy

Isotope bone scanning is a very sensitive test for assessing a loose component but is not specific. Differences between aseptic and septic loosening can only be seen if there is diffuse uptake with congruency of the early and late images. Unfortunately, not all infected prostheses show these features[1,2]. Although indium-labelled white cell imaging is better than conventional technetium scanning it does give a high incidence of false positive

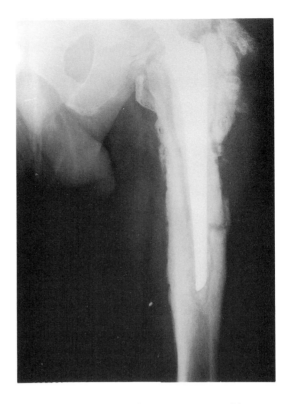

**Figure 4.1**  Loose infected femoral component with extensive periostitis.

results[3,4]. A more recent publication[5] comparing 99Tc$^m$-hexamethylpropylene-amineoxime-labelled cells with 111 inoxine-labelled cells found that the indium scans gave 37% sensitivity and the 99Tc$^m$-labelling 50% sensitivity. The conclusion from the study was that the value of labelled white scans is dependent on the activity of the infection and as most arthroplasty infections are caused by low-grade pathogens there is reduced sensitivity.

### Serology

Elevation of the erythrocyte sedimentation rate (ESR) suggests infection but unfortunately sepsis can be present with a low ESR and aseptic loosening can be associated with a high ESR. However, the ESR tends to be higher in infected than in non-infected cases. The use of C-reactive protein in conjunction with the ESR is more accurate but is also unreliable[6]. Leukergy, a phenomenon first identified in 1956, where white blood cells agglomerate in the peripheral venous blood has recently been shown to be better than any other haematological test in correlating the severity and reactivation of bone sepsis[7]. This work has not yet been applied to arthroplasty patients and further evaluation is awaited.

Other serological methods, using polyacrylamide gel electrophoresis and immunoblotting[8] have been described but again have not yet been fully evaluated.

**Table 4.1  Results of capsular biopsies**

|  | *Percentage* |
|---|---|
| Overall accuracy | 86 |
| Sensitivity | 84 |
| Specificity | 87 |
| False positive | 13 |
| False negative | 16 |

## Bacteriology

Unfortunately, there is no accurate non-invasive investigation for diagnosing infection and identifying the responsible organism. A preliminary hip aspiration and/or capsular biopsy is required. Not only is it important to identify sepsis as the reason for arthroplasty failure, it is equally imperative that both the infecting organism and its antibiotic sensitivities are known.

Many of the organisms that cause deep infection are skin commensals and great care needs to be taken when performing the aspiration to avoid contamination. Full aseptic technique is mandatory and aspiration should be performed in the operating theatre. In view of the relatively low pathogenicity of the infecting organisms, the sample should be inoculated immediately into a liquid enrichment media and transported immediately to the laboratory. Delay in arriving at the laboratory may lead to the loss of sensitive organisms and a subsequent false negative result. Contamination of the specimen may also occur in the laboratory whilst sampling for subculture. In our operating theatre, specimens are inoculated into bottles for anaerobic and aerobic culture and then promptly sent to the laboratory. We use one bottle containing brain–heart infusion broth and another with Robertson's cooked meat. The first subculture is taken on day 5 and incubated on blood agar for 48 hours, the second subculture on day 12 and again incubated for 48 hours. The bacteriology department is one of the most important factors in achieving accuracy; its members must pay particular concern to attention to detail in the various culture techniques.

The value of preoperative hip aspiration has been regarded by some[9] as an unsolved issue. We routinely aspirate and take capsular biopsies prior to revision surgery and after correlation with multiple intraoperative tissue specimens, our present results are shown in Table 4.1.

We are currently evaluating the role of capsular biopsy as this may be unnecessary as a routine if an aspirate is obtained. Biopsy should be reserved perhaps for those patients where a 'dry tap' results. Injection of isotonic saline into the joint in an attempt to wash out organisms may lead to dilution of the inoculum and false negatives may result.

Recently published results by Roberts et al.[10] using fine needle aspiration revealed a 94% accuracy, although the majority (81%) of the specimens were sterile. Barrack and Harris[9] reviewing a series of 270 consecutive hips reported an overall accuracy of 87%, 60% sensitivity and 88% specificity but again the number of proven infections at the time of revision was only 6.

The main problem with preoperative aspiration is that it is only a 'sample' and a true representation of joint contamination may not be achieved. Gristina and Costerton[11] have shown that multiple organisms may be adherent to biomaterials and therefore joint fluid may not be representative of the environment surrounding an infected implant. Less adhesive bacteria, not necessarily representative in number, type or pathogenicity of the adhesive colonies, can be shed and therefore may confuse the diagnostic picture by dominating aspirates. In addition, multiple strains of organisms with different antibiotic sensitivities, particularly *Staphylococcus epidermidis* may coexist and may not all be identified initially.

However, despite these limitations preoperative aspiration and/or capsular biopsy remain the most sensitive and specific method of diagnosing infection and is the only way of identifying the causative organism and its antibiotic sensitivities.

Gram staining of any aspirate would only identify organisms if sufficiently virulent and present in a significant concentration and therefore cannot be regarded as a reliable clinical tool.

Levitsky et al.[12] compared the value of technetium scanning, ESR > 30 and hip aspiration in the diagnosis of infection and found that aspiration was the most sensitive and specific investigation of the three (Table 4.2).

**Table 4.2  Sensitivity and specificity of preoperative diagnostic methods**

|            | Sensitivity (%) | Specificity (%) |
|------------|-----------------|-----------------|
| Technetium | 33              | 86              |
| ESR > 30   | 60              | 65              |
| Aspiration | 67              | 96              |

# Management

### Superficial sepsis

Early superficial infections such as localized cellulitis can be treated with appropriate antibiotics and local wound care. The presence of pus, however, requires surgical decompression, debridement, irrigation and antibiotic therapy. If facial planes are intact and the infection is confined to the superficial layers, then transmission to the deeper layers and to the periprosthetic tissues may not necessarily follow.

### Deep sepsis

The bacteria that colonize the infected implant live in microcolonies within biofilms that are adhesive to the surface of the prosthesis. The presence of this biofilm or glycocalyx is probably why antimicrobial therapy alone is ineffective in treating deep sepsis[11]. Any infection on a biomaterial responds poorly to antibiotic therapy and is usually not eradicated until the implant is removed.

Bacterial adherence is a positive virulence factor and may enhance protection against both antibiotics and natural host defences. It therefore follows that conservative, non-surgical management has no place in the treatment of deep sepsis. However, there are clinical instances where aggressive surgery is contraindicated, e.g. the very elderly or medically unfit patient. Here antibiotic suppression may be successful and we do have several individual cases where this has been successful.

### Acute infection

Early identification of infection within 24–48 hours of the onset of symptoms is termed acute infection and methods of treatment include intra-articular installation of antibiotic, soft-tissue debridement and parenteral antibiotic therapy. Most studies have involved knee arthroplasty as its superficial position allows an easier diagnosis of sepsis. Perry et al.[13] reported successful suppression of infection in 12 patients with a follow-up from 37 to 58

months. Their technique included drainage, amikacin intra-articular infusion for 8–15 weeks. In a larger study of 33 knee arthroplasties, treated by incision, irrigation and intravenous antibiotics, Hartman et al.[14] reported a reinfection rate of 61% after an average follow-up of 4½ years. However, presentation within 4 weeks of the onset of symptoms was associated with a more favourable outcome.

### Chronic infection

The treatment of established sepsis requires the use of basic surgical principles. Thorough debridement with removal of the implant and all involved tissues is followed by antibiotic therapy. Failure to remove all the cement from an infected arthroplasty has been shown to be associated with a significantly increased risk of failure[15]. The main objective when dealing with sepsis is to treat the infection. Reconstruction is a secondary problem and must not compromise an extensive debridement.

The concept of a resection arthroplasty was discussed by Girdlestone in 1943 for the treatment of acute pyogenic arthritis[16]. Although it is very effective for eradicating sepsis[17, 18, 19], functionally it is far from ideal as patients frequently complain of significant pain and poor ambulation, the majority requiring walking aids and built-up footwear. It is our policy in virtually all cases, to offer reconstruction following debridement either as a one- or two-stage procedure. Out of a series of 503 joint exchanges only 19 patients (4%) have been left with a permanent pseudarthrosis.

Having been shown that antibiotics elute from acrylic cement, Buchholz et al.[20] used antibiotic-loaded cement to replace an infected arthroplasty in a one-stage exchange. Others made antibiotic-laden cement beads to enhance sterilization during the interval phase in a two-stage procedure. The decision to perform either a one- or two-stage procedure depends upon several factors.

Direct exchange of an infected arthroplasty cannot be regarded as a routine procedure. Accurate bacteriology is essential and only certain infecting organisms can be dealt with in this way. It relies heavily on the concept that antibiotic can be placed in high concentration in the bone cement as a depot, subsequently leaching out locally in much greater concentrations than could be achieved by systemic infusion.

Although we have a relatively large experience with the direct exchange, we have recently become increasingly concerned with its use when dealing with coagulase-negative staphylococci and haemolytic streptococci. Different strains of coagulase-negative staphylococci often coexist with different antibiotic sensitivities and so we now think the presence of this organism is not appropriate for a single-stage exchange. Haemolytic streptococcal infections also appear rather resilient to treatment in this way. The series from the Endo Klinik[21] found no significant difference using actuarial methods in the outcome following exchange for the infections by *Staph. epidermidis*, anaerobic Corynebacterium or *Staph. aureus*. Infections caused by Pseudomonas and other Gram-negative infections produced significantly inferior results. Overall, a 77% success rate was achieved after one direct exchange, rising to 90% after further exchange procedures. Success was defined as control of infection, no loosening and useful function. These results were achieved without using systemic antibiotic therapy.

The main advantage of the direct exchange is that only one major operation is required. When the morbidity of two surgical episodes and the associated temporary pseudarthrosis are considered, the attractiveness of a direct exchange is obvious. However, more clinical failures with reinfection may occur if adequate expertise is not available. In a comparative study of the delayed versus the direct exchange, Carlsson et al.[22] reported four cases of reinfection in 18 patients having a staged procedure compared to 10 cases out of 59 direct exchanges. Unfortunately with these small numbers the results were not statistically significant.

Large doses of antibiotic powder, sometimes up to 4.5 g per 40 g polymer have been added to the cement depending upon the infecting organisms. This does not appear to have any adverse effect on the mechanical survival of the reconstruction. This is in contrast to laboratory studies where volumes greater than 2.5 g of antibiotic have been shown to have a detrimental effect on the cement's mechanical strength. In our series, the exact volume of antibiotic powder added to the cement was known in 388 cases. Fortuitously, approximately equal numbers of hips (Figure 4.2) had less than 2.5 g (184 hips: 2.5 g or less) of added antibiotic as those with greater than 2.5 (204 hips: 3–5 g) added. No statistical difference between survival in those hips with cement containing high and low antibiotic concentrations was found (Figure 4.3). However, if different age groups are studied, patients under the age of 50 years showed a higher incidence of

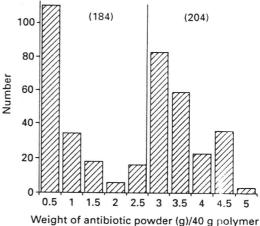

**Figure 4.2** Bar chart indicating distribution of weights of antibiotic powder added to 40g of powdered polymer before curing (Elson R. (1993) Exchange arthroplasty for infection. *Orthop. Clin. North Am.*, **24 (4)**, 761–767).

mechanical failure if high concentrations were used as compared to lower concentrations.

Uncertain bacteriology or inappropriate bacterial species and the need to bone graft for reconstruction are the main reasons for performing a two-stage procedure. Other indications include the toxic or frail patient where the patient's general poor physical state would not cope with reconstruction at the same sitting. If in doubt for whatever reason, it is safer to perform a staged procedure. The length of interval between stages is debatable varying from several weeks to over one year. Indeed, McDonald et al.[15] advise on a period of no less than 12 months before reimplantation as in their series, reinfection was significantly higher if reimplantation was undertaken within a shorter period. This has not been our experience and we try to reconstruct the hip joint after three months. A longer interval makes reconstruction more awkward as it becomes increasingly difficult to mobilize the hip in view of soft-tissue scarring.

Performing a staged procedure does allow for the endosteal surfaces of the femur and acetabulum to recover, thereby presenting a better surface for cementation with or without bone grafting.

To enhance the effectiveness of a staged procedure, antibiotic-laden polymethylmethacrylate beads can be inserted for local antibiotic delivery. Depending upon the preoperative aspiration, appropriate antibiotics can be added to the cement and an antibiotic cocktail used for maximum antimicrobial effect. By making 'home-made'

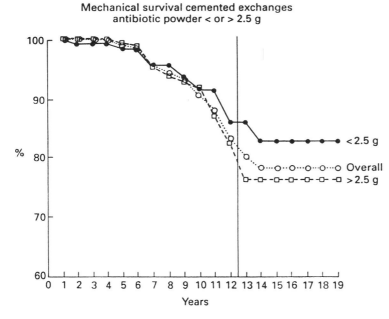

Mechanical survival cemented exchanges
antibiotic powder < or > 2.5 g

**Figure 4.3** Mechanical survival of series of exchanges with more or less than 2.5 g of antibiotic powder per 40 g polymer (Elson R. (1993) Exchange arthroplasty for infection. *Orthop. Clin. North Am.*, **24** (**4**), 761–767).

beads greater concentrations of antibiotic can be added when compared to the commercially manufactured beads (Figure 4.4). The beads are squeezed onto braided wire, flattened to enlarge the surface area and then packed into bony cavities, making every effort to avoid loose particles that could produce irritation from contact with soft tissues. Acrylic beads in contact with soft tissues can promote a very inflammatory reaction which may be extremely vascular due to the production of granulomata. Ectopic bone formation around the beads is often seen and can make dissection difficult at the time of reimplantation.

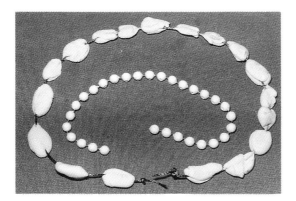

**Figure 4.4**   Home-made and commercially available methylmethacrylate beads.

After an interval, reconstruction is undertaken and again antibiotic cement can be used as an adjuvant. Different organisms may have been found at the first stage when compared to the aspiration and if necessary the antibiotic to be added to the bone cement may be changed accordingly. Aminoglycosides are the most effective antibiotics with regard to elution from the cement and so tend to be used the most. Unfortunately changing patterns of antibiotic resistance, particularly with the coagulase-negative staphylococcus has led to a search for newer antibiotic combinations. An increasing number of coagulase-negative infections are resistant to gentamicin and Hope et al.[23] have shown this to be statistically related to whether or not antibiotic-laden cement was used at the time of the primary arthroplasty. Of equal importance but not statistically significant was the fact that the failure rate due to reinfection of the subsequent exchange procedure was 8% with a gentamicin-sensitive coagulase-negative staphylococcus compared with 21% if it were gentamicin resistant.

The spectrum of the infecting organisms has changed over the years with coagulase-negative staphylococci assuming an increasing pathogenic role. This may in part be related to identification of this particular organism as over the years it has changed from being an organism of 'no note' to being a pathogen of importance in its own right. In Buchholz's series[20] the incidence of *Staph. albus* infections acting as a single infecting agent and in mixed culture was 5%. *Staph. aureus* was the most common pathogen either acting alone or in combination in 41% of cases. Fitzgerald et al.[24] and Hunter and Dandy[25] found *Staph. albus* in 27%, whereas in our series the coagulase-negative staphylococci were identified either alone or in mixed culture in 66% of cases. Thirty per cent of the coagulase-negative infections reported by Hope et al.[23] were due to multiple strains, the mechanism by which they develop being uncertain. Two possible explanations are changing antibiotic resistance in the progeny of a single parent strain and simultaneous proliferation of several different parent strains. It is important to realize that multiple strains can be present as only then can appropriate antibiotics be given. The failure rate due to reinfection after one-stage exchange was similar if single or multiple strains were present.

As an alternative to using beads and in an attempt to maintain leg length after resection arthroplasty, Duncan and Beauchamp[26] have described a custom-made, immediate fit, antibiotic-selective prosthesis. The purpose of the device being to maintain limb length, retain stability and allow elution of antibiotic, this being particularly useful when there is extensive bone loss. An additional advantage of the technique was the development of a well-vascularized channel around the prosthesis which formed a pseudocapsule in contrast to the markedly distorted scarred anatomy that one normally finds after resection arthroplasty.

## The Sheffield experience

Three factors need to be considered when evaluating the results of exchange arthroplasty for infection:

* control of infection
* mechanical survival
* radiological failure

In addition, failure may be absolute or uncertain, as there are instances when concern can arise without absolute certainty of the outcome. Recurrence of infection is sporadic, not inevitable, but when it does recur is absolute. It can therefore be measured in conventional statistics, i.e. percentages. Mechanical and radiological failure is inevitable assuming that the patient lives long enough and so can be expressed by actuarial methods.

Our documented series to date includes 503 exchange arthroplasties, 331 of which were probably infected (278 definitely infected, 53 possibly) and 172 not infected at the time of exchange. Seventy-three patients had died and 14 patients were lost to follow-up but were satisfactory at the time of last review.

The majority of operations performed were a direct exchange (79% versus 21%) reflecting traditions at the time. Failure due to infection was 15% in the series as a whole, including definite and possible failures with a four-fold increased likelihood of failure for one-stage exchanges.

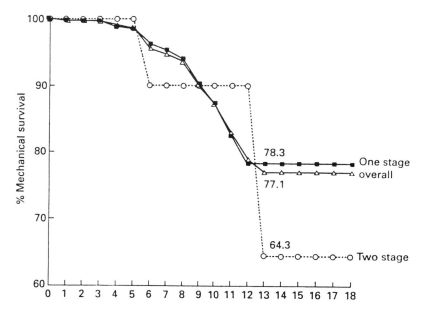

**Figure 4.5** Mechanical survival comparing overall results with those of one- and two-stage exchanges (Elson R. (1993) Exchange arthroplasty for infection. *Orthop. Clin. North Am.,* **24** (4) 761–767).

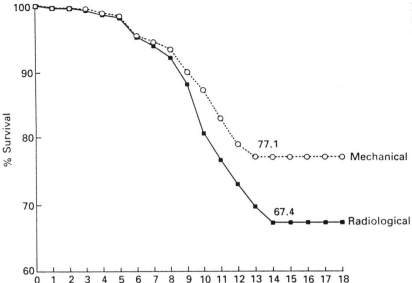

**Figure 4.6** Comparison of mechanical and radiological survivals.

Forty-three per cent of the failures were attributed to reinfection with coagulase-negative staphylococci, all having been treated by direct exchange. No reinfections of coagulase-negative staphylococci have arisen following a staged reconstruction. Mechanical survival has been alluded to previously but it should be noted again, that adding substantial quantities of extra antibiotic powder in some instances, to achieve the primary aim of eliminating infection, appears to have had no detrimental effects on the mechanical survival of the construct. Survivorship analysis of these patients (Figure 4.5) does not differ significantly from previously reported series of aseptic exchange procedures.

Radiological failure defined as progressive radiological changes of loosening without symptoms requiring surgical intervention, can be regarded as an indicator of inevitable mechanical failure and as such was more commonly found (Figure 4.6).

## Conclusions

Despite improvements in prevention, sepsis remains a substantial problem in hip arthroplasty surgery.

Prophylaxis remains the best treatment. When infection develops, exchange arthroplasty, either direct or staged, can be performed and predictable results can be obtained if accurate bacteriology is available and surgery is conducted in a specialist centre.

With regard to the future, implants should be examined to find which promote bactericidal, bacteriostatic or phagocytic activity at their surfaces and biomaterials developed to frustrate the initial adherence of bacteria that then form microcolonies. Bacteria have been around for many, many years and are highly adaptive organisms. Biomaterials are relatively new and further investigations into their own properties and behaviour are now required.

## References

1. Rushton, N., Coakley, A.J., Tudor, J. and Wraight, E.P. (1982) The value of technetium and gallium scanning in assessing pain after total hip replacement. *J. Bone Joint Surg.*, **64B**, 313–317.
2. Taylor, D.N., Maughan, J., Patel, M.P. and Clegg, J. (1989) A simple method of identifying loosening or infection of hip prostheses in nuclear medicine. *Nucl. Med. Commun.*, **10**, 551–556.
3. Pring, D.J., Henderson, R.G., Rivett, A.G. et al. (1986) Autologous granulocyte scanning of painful prosthetic joints. *J. Bone Joint Surg.*, **68B**, 647–652.
4. Magnuson, J.E., Brown, M.L., Hauser, M.F. et al. (1988) In-111-labelled leukocyte scintigraphy in suspected orthopaedic prosthesis infection: comparison with other imaging modalities. *Radiology*, **168**, 235–239.
5. Glithero, P.R., Grigoris, P., Harding, L.K. et al. (1993) White cell scans and infected joint replacements. *J. Bone Joint Surg.*, **75B**, 371–374.
6. Sanzen, L. and Carlsson, A.S. (1989) The diagnostic value of C reactive protein in infected hip arthroplasties. *J. Bone Joint Surg.*, **71B**, 638–641.
7. Otremski, I., Newman, R.J., Kahn, P.J. et al. (1993) Leukergy — A new diagnostic test for bone infection. *J. Bone Joint Surg.*, **75B**, 734–736.

8. Krickler, S.J. and Lambert, P.A. (1992) Towards a serological diagnosis of deep infection in bone. *J. Bone Joint Surg.*, **73B**, Suppl III, 316.

9. Barrack, R.L. and Harris, W.H. (1993) The value of aspiration of the hip joint before revision total hip arthroplasty. *J. Bone Joint Surg.*, **75A**; 66–76.

10. Roberts, P., Walters, A.J. and McMinn, D.J.W. (1992) Diagnosing infection in hip replacements: the use of fine needle aspiration and radiometric culture. *J. Bone Joint Surg.*, **74B**, 265–269.

11. Gristina, A.G. and Costerton, J.W. (1985) Bacterial adherence to biomaterials and tissue; the significance of its role in clinical sepsis. *J. Bone Joint Surg.*, **67A**, 264–273.

12. Levitsky, K.A., Hozack, W.J., Balderston, R.A. et al. (1991) Evaluation of the painful prosthetic joint: relative value of bone scan, sedimentation rate and joint aspiration. *J. Arthroplasty*, **6**, 237–244.

13. Perry, C.R., Hulsey, R.E., Mann, F.A. et al. (1972) Treatment of acutely infected arthroplasties with incision, drainage and local antibiotics delivered via an implantable pump. *Clin. Orthop.*, **281**, 216–223.

14. Hartman, M.B., Fehring, T.K., Jordan, L. and Norton, H.J. (1991) Periprosthetic knee sepsis — the role of irrigation and debridement. *Clin. Orthop.*, **273**, 113–118.

15. McDonald, D.J., Fitzgerald, R.H. and Ilstrup, D.M. (1989) Two stage reconstruction of a total hip arthroplasty because of infection. *J. Bone Joint Surg.*, **71A**, 828–834.

16. Girdlestone, G.R. (1943) Acute pyogenic arthritis of the hip: an operation giving free access and effective drainage. *Lancet*, **1**, 419–421.

17. Charnley, J. (1972) Postoperative infection after total hip replacement with special reference to air contamination in the operating room. *Clin. Orthop.*, **87**, 167–187.

18. Bourne, R.B., Hunter, G.A., Rorabeck, C.H. and McNab, J.J. (1984) A six year follow up of infected total hip replacements managed by Girdlestone arthroplasty. *J. Bone Joint Surg.*, **66B**, 340–344.

19. Canner, G.C., Steinberg, M.E., Heppenstall, B.R. et al. (1984) The infected hip after total hip arthroplasty. *J. Bone Joint Surg.* **66A**, 1393–1399.

20. Buchholz, H.W., Elson, R.A., Engelbrecht, E. et al. (1981) Management of deep infection of total hip replacement. *J. Bone Joint Surg.*, **63B**, 342–353.

21. Buchholz, H.W., Elson, R.A. and Heinert, K. (1984) Antibiotic loaded acrylic cement: current concepts. *Clin. Orthop.*, **190**, 96–108.

22. Carlsson, A.S., Josefsson, G. and Lindberg, L. (1978) Revision with gentamicin impregnated cement for deep infections in total hip arthroplasties. *J. Bone Joint Surg.*, **60A**, 1059–1064.

23. Hope, P.G., Kristinsson, K.G., Norman, P. and Elson, R.A. (1989) Infection of cemented hip arthroplasties by coagulase negative staphylococci. *J. Bone Joint Surg.*, **71B**, 851–855.

24. Fitzgerald, R.H. Jr, Nolan, D.R., Ilstrup, D.M. et al. (1977) Deep wound sepsis following total hip arthroplasty. *J. Bone Joint Surg.*, **59A**, 847–855.

25. Hunter, G. and Dandy, D. (1977) The natural history of the patient with an infected total hip replacement. *J. Bone Joint Surg.*, **59B**, 293–297.

26. Duncan, C.P. and Beauchamp, C. (1993) A temporary antibiotic loaded joint replacement system for management of complex infections involving the hip. *Orthop. Clin. North Am.*, **24**, 751–759.

# 5

# Tissue banking

Richard N. Villar

Tissue banking is now big business, despite the fact that the use of allograft tissue is not new. History records that it even resulted in the execution of its supposed founders, the Saints Cosmos and Damien, in AD 287[1]. However, with more than 40 000 total hip replacements being performed each year in the United Kingdom, 500 000 worldwide, failures are inevitable[2], a proportion of such failures requiring the use of bone allograft.

The creation and management of a bone bank requires great attention to detail. Though it may start out as a cottage-industry approach, very rapidly the demands placed upon it can outstrip supply. It is therefore important to cater for this eventuality at the beginning and, in particular, to ensure that a specific individual (or individuals) is appointed to handle the administration of the bone bank. Bone banking is, in essence, an accurate and demanding administrative exercise.

The creation of a bone banking service requires three things:

- Donors
- Recipients
- Somewhere to store the bone (bone bank)

## Donors

Donors may be of three types:

- Living
- Multi-organ
- Cadaver

### Living donors

Living donors are available in the greatest num-

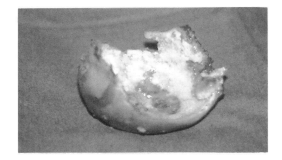

**Figure 5.1** Femoral head taken from a living donor at total hip replacement. Note the small quantity of allograft bone that such tissue provides.

bers, though the quantity of bone they can deliver is often not good (Figure 5.1). Femoral heads taken at hip replacement, or hemiarthroplasty for fractured femoral neck, are the commonest source of bone. Distal femoral and proximal tibial bone from total knee replacement can also be a reasonable source of tissue. The problem of the living donor is the quantity of administration associated with such a small volume of tissue. Despite this, living donors represent the commonest source of bone in the western world today.

### Multi-organ donors

Multi-organ donors are donors that form part of a general organ transplantation programme. Either with pre-mortem consent, or with the post-mortem permission of relatives, a number of tissues are harvested. Lungs, liver, heart, bowel, pancreas, may

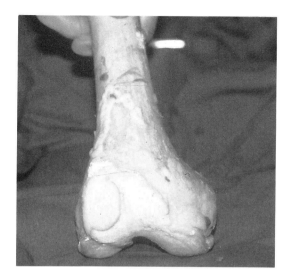

**Figure 5.2**  Massive allograft harvested from a multiorgan donor. Much larger quantities of allograft bone may be acquired from such a source.

all be obtained, bone representing a small part of the overall organ procurement. The advantage of the multi-organ donor is the large quantity of tissue that can be retrieved for a relatively modest administrative input (Figure 5.2). One such donor can provide sufficient bone for more than ten recipients, representing a very cost-effective transplantation tissue.

### Cadaver donors

Cadaver donors are very similar to multi-organ donors except that the perfused organs will not have been harvested. Such donors are likely to be harvested in the post-mortem room, again with relatives' or coroner's permission. Cadaver donors are also an excellent supply of large volumes of tissue for little administrative input.

## Ethical implications

Though tissue transplantation has been available for many years, the attitude of regular transplantation staff to bone harvesting is frequently puzzling. Nursing and paramedical staff who have been involved in heart or liver transplantation for long periods can balk at the concept of bone allografting, particularly if massive allografts are to be harvested and used. Quite why this should be so is difficult to explain, but it is vital that such staff are educated as fully as possible in the reasons that lie behind bone allografting.

Consent is vital. This should be obtained directly from the living donor, or from the donor's relatives in the case of multi-organ and cadaver donors. In these latter situations, making an approach to the relatives can be very difficult indeed. In the United Kingdom this is largely handled by Transplant Coordination Staff, individuals trained in the management of bereaved relatives and usually with a nursing qualification as well. Transplant Co-ordinators represent the mainstay of any major bone transplantation service and every effort should be made to involve them in allografting activities. They are also deeply committed to transplant education and will help spread the word of the value of musculoskeletal transplantation.

Consent should also be obtained from the allograft recipient, particularly in view of the often protracted rehabilitation that can follow such procedures. Complications of surgery are not unknown and it is wise that specific allograft consent be obtained before operation is undertaken.

## Investigations

The most important step in the elimination of disease transmission is the adoption of rigid donor exclusion criteria. In essence, any donor who is not suitable for blood transfusion is not suitable for musculoskeletal tissue donation. Medical and social screening are thus essential.

Investigation of allograft tissue and donor is therefore a vital part of musculoskeletal transplantation. At the time of harvest a small portion of bone is cultured using standard and enrichment culture for a minimum of 4 days. A further specimen is taken for culture at the time of recipient implantation, though this is optional.

The donor is tested for the following:

• Syphilis
• HIV antibodies
• Hepatitis B
• Hepatitis C

Cytomegalovirus (CMV) and toxoplasmosis are optional. Rhesus type assessment is also recommended, though not established by all tissue banks.

In the case of living donors, further HIV antibody testing should be performed at 180 days' post-harvest. This is not possible for multi-organ and cadaver donors, though an initial HIV antibody test is naturally performed in these cases.

## Storage

Allograft tissue may be used fresh, fresh frozen, or freeze-dried. Each type of tissue represents a different form of preparation and storage.

### Fresh allograft

Fresh allograft is uncommonly used at revision hip arthroplasty. The commonest reason for their use is the reconstruction of osteoarticular defects, created as a result of tumour destruction, or post-traumatic. They will not be considered here, though they do form an important part of many multi-tissue banks' activities.

### Fresh frozen allograft

Here the allograft is taken from the donor, wrapped in the appropriate layers of towelling and plastic, and placed in the bone bank. This should remain constant at the selected temperature, but normally between −23° and −80° Celsius. The frozen allograft should remain in quarantine until results of all relevant tests are available. Bone storage time is an imprecise art, but it is commonly accepted that tissue may be used for one year after storage at −23° Celsius, and up to five years when stored at −80° Celsius. Even at these lowest temperatures, freezing does not sterilize the tissue. This most definitely applies to HIV[3].

With professional tissue banking facilities, allograft bone is cleaned and defatted before banking, all surplus soft tissue being removed unless specific instructions are given for it to remain in place.

### Freeze-dried allograft

Freeze-drying (lyophilization) is an established technique, being first applied to solid human tissues in 1951[4], though reports of the technique itself appear in the literature as early as 1890. It essentially involves the dehydration of a frozen aqueous material through the sublimation of ice and is applied almost invariably to biological materials. Freeze-drying has a number of advantages. The process prevents shrinkage, chemical changes are minimized, solubility (if appropriate) is maintained, whilst the tissue may be transported and stored at room temperature. Clinically, the tissue is as effective as fresh frozen allograft when used in areas of high osteogenic capacity. However, it is not as easily handled as fresh frozen tissue and this has deterred many surgeons from using it as

routine. Immunological studies have shown that freeze-dried bone is not immunogenic, its main effect being to act as a bulk replacement, a scaffolding upon which host bone-forming cells can work. Its incorporation is said to be superior to that of frozen bone[5]. Unfortunately, freeze-dried tissue is very expensive, and is associated with a risk of collagen fibre damage. This is a significant problem for cruciate ligament allograft.

### Air-dried allograft

In a few centres, air-dried allograft is preserved. This is on the basis that lyophilization (freeze-drying) can reduce the biomechanical strength of grafts, though data concerning this are conflicting. Lyophilization of bone at freezing temperatures is not necessary to preserve the bone morphogenetic protein. The tissue may be air-dried slightly above room temperature (22–32° Celsius) without loss of osteoinductive capacity[6].

## Donor selection

Donor selection forms a vital part of tissue banking. In simple terms, criteria that would exclude an individual from being a blood donor also apply to bone donation. Regulations and recommendations are laid down by the Blood Transfusion Service, and these should be followed to the letter.

### Tissue harvest

The harvesting of bone from the living donor forms part of the normal operative procedure and will not be covered here. However, the harvesting of multi-organ and cadaver donors is a laborious procedure and can be hastened by the use of certain techniques.

The procedure should be performed in aseptic conditions if possible. In an operating theatre environment, all unnecessary personnel should be asked to leave the theatre. Bones should be exposed by longitudinal incisions straight down to bone. As much soft tissue as possible should be removed with the bone in situ (Figure 5.3). The moment the bone is removed, soft-tissue stripping becomes much harder. For femoral removal it is often easier to transect the midshaft before removing the bone, particularly if the tissue bank does not require an entire femur to be harvested. For those running their own tissue banks, it is worthwhile thinking at the time of harvest what is likely

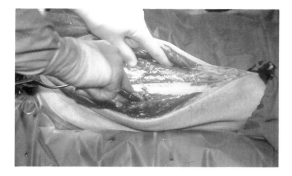

**Figure 5.3** Femoral bone harvest being performed on a multi-organ donor.

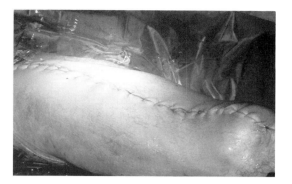

**Figure 5.4** Reconstruction is important. This multi-organ donor (see Figure 5.3) has been reconstructed with wooden dowelling rod and plaster of Paris.

to be needed for the subsequent recipient. It is a waste of bone to be given an entire femur at the time of eventual implantation, only to find that all that is required is a strut segment of the proximal shaft. Think at the time of harvest what is likely to be needed and bone wastage will be kept to a minimum.

Following bone removal, final soft-tissue stripping is performed, the tissue then being wrapped in three alternating layers of towelling and plastic. The outermost layer should be of towel as direct contact of plastic to any dry ice will result in cracking of the plastic.

The final task of any harvesting team is to record in the patient's notes exact details of the tissue removed for transplantation. This is particularly important should a subsequent post-mortem be necessary.

### Reconstruction

Reconstruction is important. The body may have to go from the operating theatre to a hospital ward, or a Chapel of Rest. It must appear to be in good condition for the sake of the relatives, or nursing staff who have never witnessed a bone harvest.

Reconstruction may be performed with wooden rods and plaster of Paris, or with special custom-made components. Both are able to be incinerated should the donor ultimately be cremated. Once limb length has been restored, the skin is closed with continuous nylon sutures (Figure 5.4) and an adhesive dressing applied.

### Recipients

Not all patients make suitable recipients of allograft bone, despite often massive loss of bone stock. Recipients should be physically strong, and emotionally strong. Physically strong because of the often prolonged crutch usage that is required after allografting procedures. Emotionally strong because of the well-recognized association between psychological changes and the receipt of transplanted tissue. It is not unusual for recipients of allograft bone, particularly massive allograft specimens, to claim they are depressed for several weeks after the procedure.

### Bone bank

A bone bank is essentially a sophisticated freezer. Its aim is to preserve musculoskeletal tissue for as long as is safe and practical.

In many hospitals, the bone bank is to be found within the theatre complex, often supervised by a member of theatre staff on a part-time or voluntary basis. It is perfectly possible to run a banking system in such a way, but it invites problems. Better control is obtained if at least one member of staff is dedicated to the task of running the bone bank, and is made responsible for the collation of all results, sterilization of tissue, security and general administration. This is a difficult and time-consuming task.

A bone bank should be fitted with a continuous temperature recorder and alarm that sounds whenever the temperature falls below a preset value, or when the electricity supply fails. It should also be locked, the key being held by specific, allocated individuals. Access should be denied to all except these chosen few. Only in this way can contamination and cross-infection be controlled.

Within the bank itself, a specific area should be set aside for tissue in quarantine, awaiting the HIV status, and bacteriological results of the donors. It should then be moved to a different area of the bank once it is available for use.

A log book should be created that will allow all relevant details of donor and recipient to be seen at a glance. This should also be kept under lock and key and be the only document where donor and recipient can be connected. Such details should not be kept in the recipient's notes. However, consent forms, and the bone bank number may be kept in the notes. If required, the bone bank log book may be computerized, an invaluable asset for a large, multi-tissue bank that may be serving a number of hospitals and regions. Even if tissue be sent to a hospital overseas, it is essential the bank administrator be aware of the recipient of the tissue, for effective audit purposes.

## Sterilization of allograft

The moment a musculoskeletal allograft is introduced into a recipient, an infection risk exists. Lord et al.[7] reported an 11.7% infection rate in 283 patients who had received massive allografts for tumour reconstruction. The majority of infections were caused by *Staph. epidermidis* with 82% of infected allografts requiring amputation. This research did not involve femoral head allografts, nor soft-tissue allografts, but it is none the less not surprising that allografting has developed an image of being infection-prone. It is probable that the infection rate associated with the smaller allografts is actually negligible, whilst the rate for massive allograft usage at revision hip replacement is of the order of 4%.

Studies also exist of the infection rates following massive prosthetic replacement, with a wide variety of results from 0 to 11%. It is probable therefore that the cause of infection following allograft surgery is not the use of the allograft, but the nature of the surgery involved. Long operating times, wide soft-tissue exposures, multiple surgeons, and so on.

None the less, there is no room for complacency. Contamination of allografts is a genuine risk, with rates of more than 30%[8] being reported. To a large extent the contamination rate of a bone bank

is proportional to the enthusiasm of its microbiological back-up. Without a dedicated, interested bacteriologist it is quite usual to find very low contamination rates. In the presence of enthusiastic microbiological support, 30% contamination can actually appear quite reasonable. Reports from the Netherlands have highlighted contamination rates of 58% of specimens extracted under sterile conditions from cadaveric donors. It is for this reason that many professionally-run tissue banks rely on secondary sterilization of tissue. Not all do so, however. The risk of transmission of disease, particularly viral infection, depends largely on the prevalence of infectious carriers, and any precautions taken to eliminate material from these donors[9]. Hepatitis B virus, for example, can survive freeze-drying and freezing/thawing[10]. Human immunodeficiency virus (HIV) has been transferred to patients receiving kidney, heart, liver, skin, and bone transplantation[11]. Other viral worries include Creutzfeldt–Jakob disease, and even rabies. Both have been transmitted via corneal transplantation. Creutzfeldt-Jakob has also been transmitted via freeze-dried dura that had been both irradiated and ethylene oxide-sterilized[12].

Rhesus compatibility is also advisable, as only 0.5 ml of red blood cells is required to immunize a Rhesus-negative recipient[13].

There are a number of different methods of sterilizing allograft. These are:

1. Heat
2. Ethylene oxide
3. Irradiation
4. Surface cleaning
5. Miscellaneous methods (see below)

### Heat

Heat sterilization has long been accepted as a method of sterilizing bone allografts, first proposed at the turn of this century. A number of authors have since reported on their clinical experiences with autoclaved grafts, though mainly in tumour surgery. Chiron et al.[14] suggested that autoclaving of allograft bone resulted in a complete disappearance of bone marrow, though the trabecular bone remained intact macroscopically. Bone in this study was heated to 120° Celsius for 20 minutes. The authors' final conclusion was that autoclaving did not alter the structure of the bone and was thus a safe, cost-effective method of sterilization. What is unquestionably true, however, is that at temperatures above 60° Celsius, protein is coagulated and bone morphogenetic protein is thus destroyed. A lesser osteogenic response is thus the result[15].

Other studies, however, would disagree, suggesting that autoclaving reduces the mechanical performance of allograft bone significantly and would therefore advocate it for restricted use only[16]. The complication rate with autoclaved allograft bone has also been regarded as quite high, as much as 17% in some cases. However, work has suggested that the response of bone to autoclaving is in part proportional to the temperature to which it has been exposed. A waterbath at 65° Celsius is able to inactivate viruses, and yet have no major biological effects on the bone.

### Ethylene oxide

Ethylene oxide is widely used as a sterilizing agent in musculoskeletal transplantation. It poses two worries. First, does the gas penetrate the allograft sufficiently to inactivate organisms in the very centre of the bone allograft sample? Second, are toxic materials left behind that may be to the detriment of the patient? Work has been done at the Yorkshire (UK) Tissue Bank to suggest that there is, in fact, a 6-fold overkill by ethylene oxide and that toxic residuals are not left behind. Though allegedly non-toxic, work from the Netherlands has suggested that the substance may reduce the osteo-inductive potential of allograft bone.

### Irradiation

Irradiation is perhaps the simplest method of sterilizing allograft bone, provided the tissue bank has access to an irradiation plant. Gamma-irradiation is more effective than beta-irradiation due to its better penetration, though several hours are necessary for tissue sterilization. Viruses are largely more radioresistant than bacteria. Most banks expose tissue to 25 kiloGrays (kGy) of irradiation, though 15kGy is all that is required to inactivate HIV. Irradiation has also been shown to reduce the mechanical performance of allograft bone, in particular compressive stiffness and elasticity, both of which are reduced by some 50% following irradiation. This is similar to the reduction in mechanical performance following autoclavation. It has also been shown to inactivate the bone morphogenetic protein[17], though the destructive effect of radiation is probably greater on freeze-dried tissue than on fresh frozen allograft.

None the less, the clinical results of irradiated bone allografts appear to be good, with clinical success rates as high as 85% being reported[18].

### Surface cleaning

The concern over the effects of irradiation and ethylene oxide on bone, or perhaps the expense, has led some workers to investigate the effects of surface cleaning as a sterilizing agent. Chloroform, povidone-iodine, or a high pressure water jet have been studied. These methods have been shown to reduce the micro-organism count by 80–90%, though the remainder grow exponentially thereafter. Thus, as a sole method of sterilization, surface cleaning is inadequate, but as a supplementary method it is good. Many orthopaedic units would therefore use surface cleaning at the time of surgery, as a boost to previous sterilizing methods that have been used by the supplying tissue bank. This is particularly appropriate in massive allografting, when graft preparation time can be lengthy, and intra-operative contamination a genuine risk.

### Miscellaneous methods

Many other methods of allograft sterilization have been tried, with varying success rates. These include formaldehyde, glutaraldehyde, ethyl alcohol, merthiolate, cialit, silver nitrate, benzalkonium, β-propriolactone, and hydrochloric acid.

## Tissue bank policy

It is said that in the United States of America, more than 300 000 musculoskeletal allografts are transplanted annually. In Germany, 25 000 grafts are transplanted. In one tissue bank alone, in Berlin, 50 000 grafts have been supplied to more than 250 hospitals over 35 years. Similar banks are in operation worldwide, and yet no common policy has been developed. In the United Kingdom a large number of small bone banks exist, largely in support of individual orthopaedic departments. And yet policies vary from those banks that consent neither donor nor recipient and avoid the use of HIV tests as routine, to those who discard all bone found to be contaminated, preferring not to undertake secondary sterilization procedures.

Because of such diversity of opinion, a number of tissue bank policies have been developed, some supported by force of law, others not. Such policies cover the general organizational requirements of a tissue bank, the acquisition of tissues, retrieval, processing, preservation, and storage[19]. In the United Kingdom no official policies exist, though the British Orthopaedic Association, in conjunction with the Department of Health, has produced recommended guidelines for all bone banks to follow.

Whether a bone bank should make a financial charge for its tissue is again an emotive subject. Particularly so in those countries that do not pay the donor for tissue acquired. In the United Kingdom allograft tissue is largely provided free of charge, though payment is requested for the services involved in its preparation. In this way ethical standards are maintained.

## The future

Musculoskeletal allografting has made an enormous contribution to orthopaedic surgery, but there is no doubt that it carries with it certain risks, risks common to all major operations, and the risk of disease transmission if guidelines are not followed. The day of the small, cottage-industry bone bank is now almost over. Bone banking is a task for professional, committed staff, trained in organ preservation. However, bone substitutes may be the way forward. Allograft is useful, providing a highly biocompatible, almost custom-made material for use at surgery. None the less, bone substitutes carry with them few risks and may, in time, provide a favourable alternative.

## References

1. Mankin, H.J., Doppelt, S. and Tomford, W. (1983) Clinical experience with allograft implantation: the first ten years. *Clin. Orthop.*, **174**, 69–86.
2. Villar, R. (1992) Failed hip replacements. *Br. Med. J.*, **304**, 3–4.
3. Buck, B.E., Resnick, L., Shah, S.M. and Malnin, L. (1990) Human immunodeficiency virus cultured from bone. *Clin. Orthop.*, **251**, 249–253.
4. Kruetz, F.P., Hyatt, G.W., Turner, T.C. and Bassett, A.J. (1951) The preservation and clinical use of freeze-dried bone. *J. Bone Joint Surg.*, **33A**, 863–872.
5. Heiple, K.G., Chase, S.W. and Herndon, C.H. (1963) A comparative study of the healing process following different types of bone transplantation. *J. Bone Joint Surg.*, **45A**, 1593–1616.
6. McCullough, J. and Eastlund, D.T. (1991) Tissue and organ preservation and transplantation. In *Principles of Transfusion Medicine* (E.C. Rossi, T.L. Simon, and G.S. Moss, eds) Baltimore: Williams & Wilkins, p. 677.
7. Lord, C.F., Gebhardt, M.C., Tomford, W.W. and Mankin, H.J. (1988). Infection in bone allografts: incidence, nature, and treatment. *J. Bone Joint Surg.*, **70A(3)**, 369–376.
8. Chapman, P.G. and Villar, R. (1992) The bacteriology of bone allografts. *J. Bone Joint Surg.*, **74B**, 398–399.
9. Angermann, P. and Jepsen, O.B. (1991) Procurement banking and decontamination of bone and collagenous tissue allografts: guidelines for infection control. *J. Hosp. Infect.*, **17(3)**, 159–169 (83 ref).
10. Doppelt, S.H., Tomford, W.W., Lucas, A.D. and Mankin, H.J. (1981) Operational and financial aspects of a hospital bone bank. *J. Bone Joint Surg.*, **63A**, 1472–1481.
11. Transmission of HIV through bone transplantation: Case report and public health recommendations (1988) *Morbidity and Mortality Weekly Report*, **37**, 597–599 Reported in (*JAMA*, 1988 **260**, 2487–2488).
12. Pritchard, J., Thadani, V., Kalb, R. et al. (1982) Rapidly progressive dementia in a patient who received a cadaveric dura mater graft. *Morbidity and Mortality Weekly Report* **35**, 49–55.
13. Mollison, P.L. (1983) Post-transfusion viral hepatitis. In *Blood Transfusion in Clinical Medicine* (P.L. Morrison, ed.) Oxford: Blackwell Scientific Publications, pp. 768–774.
14. Chiron, Ph, Gaudy, E., Utheza, G. et al. (1992) Heat sterilization of bone allografts. European Association of Musculoskeletal Transplantation, April (Abstract) 10.
15. Prolo, D.J., Pedrotti, P.W. and White, D.H. (1980) Ethylene oxide sterilization of bone, dura mater, and fascia lata for human transplantation. *Neurosurg.* **6**, 529–539.
16. Garrel, T., Knaepler, H., Seipp, H-M. et al. (1991) Experimental and clinical experiences with autoclaved allogenic bone grafts (abstract). First European Conference on Tissue Banking. 36.
17. Buring, K. and Urist, M.R. (1967) Effects of ionizing radiation on the bone induction principle in the matrix of bone implants. *Clin. Orthop.*, **55**, 25–234.
18. Bassett, C.A.L. and Packard, A.G. (1959) A clinical assay of cathode ray sterilized cadaver bone grafts. *Acta Orthop. Scand.*, **28**, 198–211.
19. European Association of Musculoskeletal Transplantation for Tissue Banking and Current Developments (1994). Standards for Tissue Banking. EAMST.

# 6

# Treatment options

Graham S. Keene and Richard N. Villar

## Introduction

Treatment options for revision hip arthroplasty (Table 6.1) are influenced by the underlying pathology necessitating revision and the age of the patient. Naturally the expectations of a young man requiring revision surgery differ greatly from those of an elderly lady who may place lower demands on the revision. The increasing age of our population, coupled with a tendency to offer arthroplasty at a younger age, could theoretically lead to a dramatic increase in the number of patients requiring revision hip surgery in the next few years. The overall revision rate for implant loosening within 10 years of primary arthroplasty is around 10%, but may be higher in certain groups — 30% in young males[1].

The long-term results of revision hip surgery may not be as durable and gratifying as the long-term results of primary hip arthroplasty[2–5]. More scar tissue is generated, mobility may be compromised, bone stock has been lost by the process of osteolysis and must be restored. Revision surgery is also more complicated than primary surgery — a wider range of equipment is required, the blood loss is greater, the surgery more extensive and time consuming. The risks of nerve damage, shaft fracture, initial instability, infection, thromboembolic phenomenon etc. are higher.

One explanation for these disappointing long-term results, at least for cemented components, may relate to fixation at the cement–bone interface. As bone stock is lost, the trabeculated bone surface becomes smooth. This leads to a poor interference fit, as there are fewer crevices available for mechanical interlock with cement. The maximum interface shear strength between cement and bone after revision surgery has been estimated from an *in vitro* study to be 20.6% of the strength achieved at primary arthroplasty[6]. This is reduced further to 6.8% of the primary strength following a second revision. Third generation pressurized cementing techniques may lead to some improvement in these figures.

**Table 6.1  Treatment options for revision hip arthroplasty**

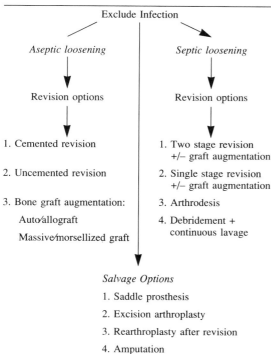

These results and the recognition that bone stock must be restored, has stimulated use of uncemented components, combined with bone graft if required. Early encouraging results of cementless revision arthroplasties are reported[7–15], although follow-up is relatively short.

The more frequently used techniques for revision hip arthroplasty are described in detail in this book, together with an indication of the long-term outcome. Although many of the possible treatment options available are discussed in this chapter, the emphasis is upon those techniques not discussed extensively elsewhere.

Revision surgery must be addressed from two aspects — the acetabular component and the femoral component. Naturally if one component can be left undisturbed, the complexity of the procedure is eased and the morbidity may be reduced. Attempts should be made to find suitable components of matching dimensions — this has been simplified with the introduction of modular prostheses. In the presence of infection, a two-stage revision procedure may be preferable.

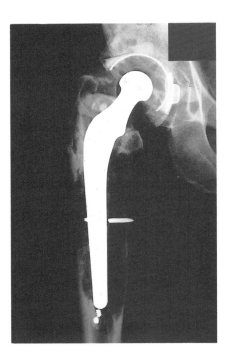

**Figure 6.1**   A loose total hip replacement.

## Indications for revision

There are two principal indications for revision (Table 6.2) — aseptic loosening (Figure 6.1) and infection (Figure 6.2). Relative indications include progressive loss of bone stock and recurrent dislocation. In the past, stem fracture was a further indication — with modern manufacturing techniques, this complication is seldom experienced. In broad terms, the treatment options are especially influenced by the presence or absence of infection, and the degree of bone stock loss. In the presence of longstanding infection, there may be considerable loss of bone stock.

The use of bone graft is often desirable with revision surgery. Bone graft may be either morsellized or block graft — 'struts' ('patch') or 'massive'. The graft may be obtained from the patient — autograft, or transplanted — allograft. Large

**Table 6.2   Principal and relative indications for revision arthroplasty**

| Indications: | Principal | Aseptic loosening |
| --- | --- | --- |
|  |  | Septic loosening |
|  | Relative | Progressive loss of bone stock |
|  |  | Recurrent dislocation |
|  |  | Component failure |

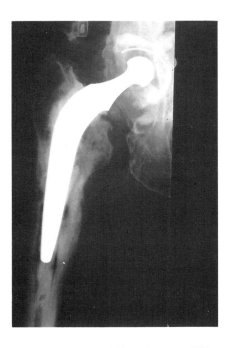

**Figure 6.2**   An infected total hip replacement. Without further investigation, these may be difficult to distinguish.

sections of block autograft are rarely feasible to obtain and allograft from the bone bank is used as a substitute.

Excision arthroplasty is often considered a last option for revision surgery. The value of excision arthroplasty should not be underestimated at the expense of attempting an extensive revision procedure. It will at least save the patient prolonged surgery, and associated mortality and morbidity, should the revision fail at an early stage.

## Preoperative planning

In common with all surgery, preoperative planning is essential. For revision surgery, planning plays a particularly important role, although the intraoperative findings and potential complications may lead to an alteration from the original plan. Good quality radiographs of the pelvis and entire femur, both in the anteroposterior and lateral planes are required. Details of the existing prosthesis should be obtained, as dedicated instrumentation may be required, and the head size should be determined so appropriate components are available in advance.

Although one component may clearly show features of failure on plain radiographs, the other component may appear sound. A $^{99m}$technetium methylene-diphosphonate (MDP) isotope bone scan may reveal unexpected loosening of both components. The presence of infection should always be considered (Figure 6.3) and baseline investigations including a full blood count, an erythrocyte sedimentation rate and C-reactive protein levels are mandatory before undertaking revision surgery.

The occasional finding of intrapelvic migration of the acetabular cup may warrant a computerized tomogram, and possibly contrast enhanced angiograms and ureterograms, preoperatively.

## Surgical approach

Revision surgery may be performed through any of the approaches used for a primary procedure; the approach with which the surgeon is familiar being the most appropriate. There are proponents of every approach, who argue the most favourable access. The skin incision should involve as much of the old scar as possible, however, the skin around the hip is well vascularized and necrosis between 'tram-lines' is rarely a problem.

As greater access is desirable for revision surgery, a more extensive exposure is required. Where modular components have been used and the original femoral component can be preserved, access may be facilitated by removing the femoral head. Alternatively, the femoral component may be extracted and reinserted[16] if the acetabulum alone requires revision.

Good exposure and access to the proximal femur is a prerequisite for cement removal and may be easier with the patient in the lateral decubitus position. Access can be improved with a trochanteric osteotomy. However, wiring is required to reattach the trochanter, which often fails to unite. This may be painful and wire removal is sometimes necessary.

An alternative approach was developed by McMinn et al.[17] — a V-shaped myofascial flap of the proximal part of vastus lateralis and its fascia, together with gluteus medius and minimus is reflected off the greater trochanter and proximal femur. This greatly improves access to the capsule and exposure of the acetabulum. Where limb

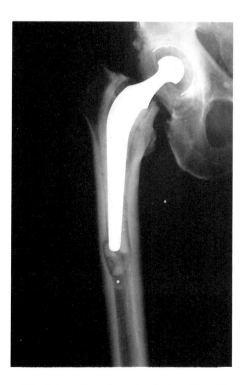

**Figure 6.3** A loose Charnley arthroplasty, with a nidus of infection at the lower pole of the femoral component. The acetabular cup appears sound.

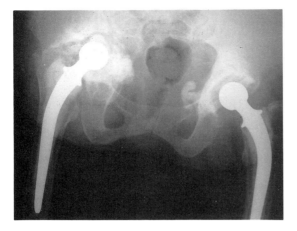

**Figure 6.4**   An acetabular cup, with intrapelvic migration.

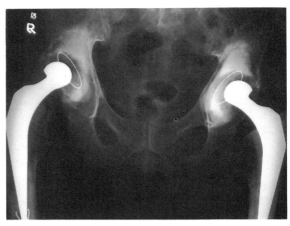

**Figure 6.5**   Bilateral acetabular loosening and loss of bone stock in a 47-year-old male, many years after primary surgery. The femoral component appears sound.

length has been restored during revision, the abductor tension can be adjusted by altering the reattachment of the flap to form a V–Y plasty.

Where the acetabular cup has migrated into the pelvis (Figure 6.4), retrieval can be hazardous, as major vascular and urological structures may be adjacent to the cup, although a layer of fibrous tissue usually distinguishes the cup from vital structures. It may even be difficult to dislocate such a hip. A simple technique for the exposure of an intrapelvic cup or cement mass has been described by Grigoris et al.[18]. Subperiosteal elevation of iliacus and medial retraction of iliopsoas exposes the cup which is retrieved by developing the plane between the polyethylene and the surrounding fibrous layer.

## The acetabulum

Deficiency of pelvic bone stock is a major challenge in the revision of a failed arthroplasty. Initial loss of bone stock may be related to the primary pathology and surgery. Further loss may be secondary to wear products and motion between bone and prosthesis, or bone and cement (Figure 6.5). The greater the loss of bone stock, the harder it becomes to achieve secure fixation of the new implant, in a biomechanically optimal position, to provide long-term stability.

Acetabular bone deficiencies have been classified by D'Antonio et al.[19]. The majority of failures have a mild or moderate deficiency which may

be Type I — segmental, Type II — cavitatory, or Type III — combined. Where the loss of bone stock from the acetabulum is minimal, Type I and Type II deficiencies, yet the prosthesis is loose, the acetabulum can be revised with a cemented component.

There are few reports relating specifically to the use of uncemented acetabular components for revision surgery. Pre-existing pathology may have resulted in a degree of disuse osteoporosis which may jeopardize the incorporation of an uncemented component. Padgett et al.[15] report successful early results in 129 uncemented porous titanium mesh hemispherical coated acetabular cups. Fixation was augmented with screws and acetabular defects were generally enlarged to accept a larger cup, maximizing bone–host contact. In 80% of cases bone autograft or allograft was used. Of this series, only 5% of the acetabular cups required revision in the first 44 months and there were no cases of aseptic loosening. Engh et al.[10] revealed a 42% migration rate at 4.4 years for acetabular revision using a threaded cup. The results of hemispherical acetabular cups, allowing bony ingrowth are generally superior to threaded cups.

Where bone stock loss is greater, this must be replaced. In the presence of a relatively small deficiency, a morsellized or block autograft will suffice. If the defect is larger, morsellized or block allograft will be required. Uncemented acetabular prostheses do not incorporate well with massive allograft blocks and cemented fixation is recommended.

If morsellized graft is being used, the acetabulum should be prepared and all debris and loose material curetted out, to leave a healthy, preferably bleeding, raw bone surface. The morsellized graft is impacted on the prepared acetabular bed, using an appropriately-sized acetabular trial or sizing instrument. The acetabular cup is then cemented on the impacted graft (Figure 6.6), using a pressurization technique, taking care not to dislodge the graft.

An alternative technique is to use a large block allograft, augmented with morsellized autograft or allograft. A femoral head serves as very suitable bone. The block is held in place with screws and morsellized graft packed around prior to cementing the acetabular cup with pressurized bone cement.

In the presence of a massive acetabular deficiency, further support for the graft may be achieved with an acetabular reinforcement 'ring' or 'cage'. A reinforcement ring provides a bridge between the host bone and acetabular cup, protecting the bone graft from excessive strain whilst incorporation of the bone graft ensues. The acetabular cup is secured by cementing to the reinforcement ring. A number of reinforcement rings are commercially available. Berry and Müller[20] report a success rate of greater than 75% in a series of 42 patients using the Burch–Schneider anti-protrusio cage, with a mean follow-up of five years. Similarly, Rosson and Schatzker[21] recommend the use of the Müller ring for peripheral segmental defects, and the Burch–Schneider cage for larger and medial defects, with a failure rate of less than 8% at five years. The use of bone graft to enhance bone stock restoration was favoured in preference to large volumes of cement. Figur 6.7 shows progressive reconstitution of pelvic bone stock with a reinforcement cage and morsellized allograft, in a case with advanced loss of acetabular bone stock.

A novel alternative to reconstruct a grossly deficient acetabulum has been developed by McMinn[22]. The principle is to pack morsellized bone graft around a long-stemmed acetabular component. The iliopubic bar of the pelvis provides support for the long stem of the acetabular component, whilst the conical cup acts as a scaffold around which morsellized graft is packed. Early results suggest reconstitution of the deficient acetabular bone stock.

## Femoral shaft

The femoral shaft is more frequently the site of greater bone stock loss which must be addressed. Being predominantly cancellous bone, the proximal femur has a fine cortical layer. As bone stock is eroded, a cavitatary defect is created. There may be healthy cancellous, trabeculated bone beyond this, to which a secure cement interference fit can be achieved, perhaps with a larger prosthesis. Alternatively, morsellized bone graft may be impacted around an uncemented or cemented prosthesis.

Femoral defects may be of various types. There may be a relatively small 'window' within the cortex. If this is less than 30% the reduction in strength of the femur is not significant and the defect may be filled with cement, or augmented with graft. It is, however, wise to bridge the defect with the replacement prosthesis, to prevent the development of a stress riser, which would predispose to a fracture.

Larger defects require an onlay strut ('patch') graft — usually an allograft, appropriately tailored to match the host femur, secured with cerclage wires. The host–graft interface should be augmented with morsellized cancellous bone graft — donor, or preferably host.

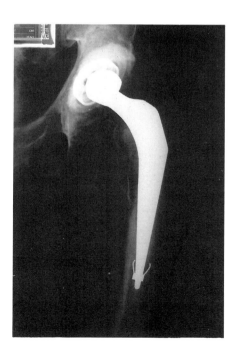

**Figure 6.6** Acetabular revision with impacted morsellized allograft, Figure 6.5 two months after revision.

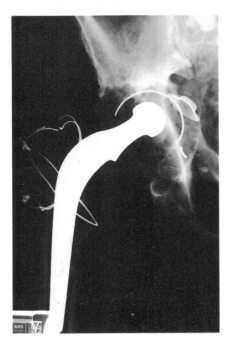

(a)

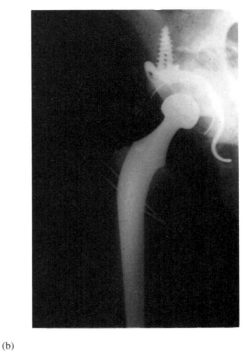

(b)

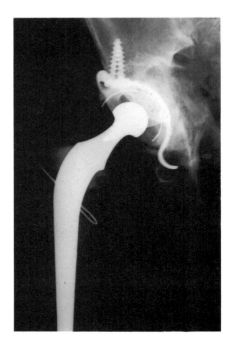

(c)

(d)

**Figure 6.7**   There is progressive reconstitution of acetabular bone stock following revision of a grossly deficient acetabulum a, using a reinforcement cage and morsellized allograft; b, 3 months postoperatively; c, 6 months postoperatively; d, 12 months postoperatively and e, 2 years postoperatively.

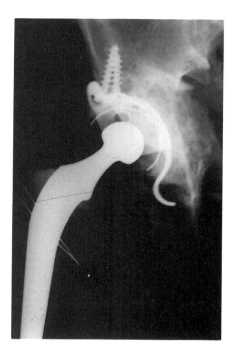

(e)

Where cavitatary and cortical defects are combined, much of the proximal femur may be weakened and deficient. If bone is preserved below the level of the lesser trochanter, a special calcar-replacing revision prosthesis may be used. In some cases, however, loss of bone stock is often advanced and the sole remaining option is a massive femoral allograft, from the tissue bank — either strut allografts or a proximal femoral replacement.

### Cemented femoral revision

In selected patients, where the components are loose, yet bone stock is well preserved, a cemented revision may be undertaken, without resorting to the more complex procedure of bone grafting. When the prosthetic head is of an unusual size, yet the acetabular component is sound, it may even be possible to recement the original femoral component. The wisdom of revising one component may be doubtful[23] especially in younger patients, as loosening of the undisturbed component may occur at an early stage after surgery.

Particular attention should be paid to preparation of the femoral shaft. The old bone cement should be removed and the associated debris curetted from the canal — the integrity of the femoral canal must be preserved. After thorough cleaning,

scrubbing, lavage and drying, the prosthesis should be secured with pressurized bone cement.

It is accepted that the results of cemented revision arthroplasty are inferior to the results of primary hip arthroplasty[2,4,5]. Infection rates are higher, aseptic loosening is more frequent and prone to occur earlier. The bone cement interface is weaker[6]. Many reported results are of a relatively short follow-up, yet high failure rates are substantial. Kershaw et al.[24] considered their results to be good. Pain was minimal in 83% and greater than half could walk a mile or more, in a series of 220 cemented revision hip arthroplasties for aseptic loosening, followed for a mean of 75 months. However, in this period, 18 patients required further surgery and 6 more cases were radiologically and symptomatically loose. Strömberg et al.[25] reported poor results from a multicentre clinical review. In a series of 204 revisions, loosening occurred in 38% of hips over 7 years and the survival rate, with re-revision as an end point, was estimated to be 75% at 8 years. Engelbrecht et al.[23] reported better results with a 7.4 year follow-up study of 138 cases of revision hip arthroplasty. There was evidence of radiological loosening in some 40% of cases, although the revision rate was 8.8% over this period. In a series of 162 hips 9% required a second revision during the 4.5 year study period reported by Kavanagh and Fitzgerald[2].

After revision surgery a radiolucent halo may be seen at the bone–cement interface. Pellicci et al.[26] found an increased failure rate with long-term follow-up of revision hip arthroplasties. Progressive and circumferential radiolucent defects at the cement–bone interface indicated a poor prognosis. Correlation between radiographic changes, loosening and pain was poor.

### Uncemented femoral revision

The femoral prosthesis may be replaced with an uncemented prosthesis, secured by means of a good press-fit. To achieve a good fit, reasonable bone stock must be available. There are few results in the literature of accurate long-term results following uncemented revision; 160 cementless revisions followed for 4.4 years by Engh et al.[10] showed optimal femoral fixation in 84.3% of cases. In a review of 56 cases by Lord et al.[8] 70% of patients were found to have satisfactory results following cementless revision. Morrey and Kavanagh[14] report a high incidence of stem failure and early subsidence with uncemented femoral components. Their early clinical assessment of uncemented and cemented revisions was broadly comparable. Harris et al.[12] and Hedley et al.[9] report encouraging early results, although the follow-up periods were short. A prosthesis designed to effectively 'fill' the proximal femur may reduce the complications of subsidence and loosening, by allowing better contact with the bone surface, so preventing proximal stress shielding.

## Bone allografting

### Strut allograft revision

Where the bone stock deficiency is advanced, but not necessarily circumferential, the cortical shell may be augmented with struts of bone allograft, appropriately fashioned for the host femur. If a transfemoral approach is used, this has the advantage of leaving an envelope of biologically active host bone around the allograft, which will augment the incorporation process. The strut allografts are secured with stout cerclage wires, the replacement prosthesis usually being uncemented (Figure 6.8). A good press-fit into the femur distal to the deficiency can usually be achieved. Morsellized autograft should be packed around the struts, especially at the host–graft interface, to promote incorporation.

Healing, or union, of strut allografts is by a process of rounding off at the end of the strut as early callus formation forms partial bridging between the host and allograft. As this consolidates, complete bridging occurs. The repair process results in the remodelling of the host femur and to some extent the allograft. Finally the strut blends to the host bone, increasing the overall bone stock.

Emerson et al.[27], in a review of 114 revision hip arthroplasties requiring strut allografts, report a consistent and reliable union rate of 8.4 months. Union rates were 96.6%, with minimal resorption of the strut allograft. Similarly encouraging results are reported by Chandler and Penenberg[28].

### Massive allograft revision

In cases where osteolysis has been aggressive and the majority of the proximal femur has been resorbed, the only practical way bone stock and function restoration can be achieved is by augmenting the proximal femur with a 'massive' allograft, and a long-stem prosthesis to bridge the defect. The allograft, replacing the proximal femur, is prepared by a second surgical team. The pros-

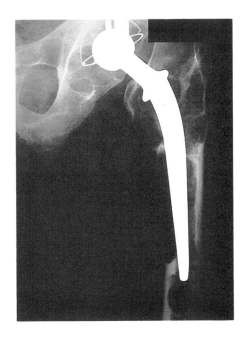

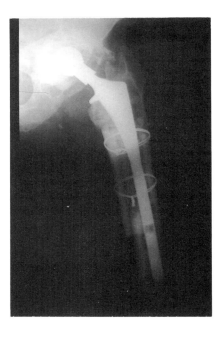

**Figure 6.8**   A loose total hip replacement, revised with an uncemented femoral component, augmented by strut allograft.

thesis should be secured to the allograft with bone cement as bone ingrowth, even to a coated implant, will not occur. In addition, although one may achieve a good interference fit in the operating theatre, there is likely to be some softening and resorption of the bone in the early postoperative phase, which will compromise any press-fit, initially perceived to be secure. Accordingly the prosthesis should be cemented to the allograft and then inserted as a combined construct, after prior trial reduction to confirm correct graft and leg length.

The distal pole of the revision prosthesis may be uncemented and secured with a good interference fit. The press fit may be augmented with interlocking screws[29]. Alternatively, the distal pole may be secured to the femur with pressurized bone cement.

Rotational stability of the graft/prosthesis construct must also be achieved. This is accomplished with a step cut, matched between the allograft construct and proximal end of the remaining host femur. The junction should be reinforced with cerclage wiring and morsellized autograft at the host-donor interface, to maximize the biological potential for union.

Again, the remnant of the proximal host femur should be wrapped around the massive allograft, secured with cerclage wires. This will augment the incorporation process. The soft tissues and cortical shell are biologically active and become attached to the allograft. This reduces stress on the construct and promotes union.

Allan et al.[30] report a series of 78 revision hip arthroplasties, all requiring bone allografts for significant defects. An 85% success rate is reported for massive femoral allografts and 86% success rate for strut allografts. There was an incidence of less than 8% unstable non-unions following massive femoral allografting. It is interesting to note the magnitude of revision surgery in the face of diminishing bone stock — 83% of their series also required an acetabular allografting procedure.

Primary union rates for massive allografts are slower than allograft struts and of course considerably slower than union rates with autograft. The healing, or bonding, to the host bone is by a process known as creeping substitution[31] generating a biological weld at the host-graft interface. Where an unstable non-union occurs, treatment by internal fixation and autogenous bone grafting will frequently precipitate biological welding. Figure 6.9 shows excellent incorporation of a massive femoral allograft 4 years after revision surgery.

There is little value in bone grafting relatively small defects around the calcar as results are disappointing — 'napkin ring' allografts for defects less than 3 cm tend to be resorbed[30]. In these

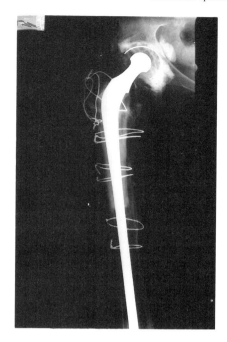

**Figure 6.9** Incorporation of a massive proximal femoral allograft, 4 years after revision. Note the remodelling at the host–graft interface.

situations it is preferable to sacrifice some leg length, or use a calcar-replacing prosthesis and secure a sound fixation within the remainder of the femoral shaft, provided adequate tissue tension to prevent dislocation can be achieved.

### Impaction grafting

An alternative to the massive replacement of the proximal femur is to augment the femoral remnant shell with impacted morsellized cancellous bone graft. This technique has been developed and refined in Exeter and the Netherlands[32] and early results were reported by Gie et al.[33]. The principle is to impact morsellized cancellous bone allograft into the femoral canal, the circumference of which is maintained by the remnant femoral shell. With vigorous impaction it is possible to achieve an impressive degree of stability of the trial stem.

Special instrumentation is required to ensure the neomedullary canal which is created, remains central within the host femur. The replacement prosthesis is cemented onto the impacted allograft with low viscosity, pressurized, bone cement. This is a modification of the technique promoted by Slooff et al.[34] for revision of the deficient acetabulum.

In 1990 Nelson et al.[35] reported 3 cases of impaction allograft augmented with a cortico-cancellous iliac crest autograft, to reconstruct the proximal femur. The two-year results, with an uncemented prosthesis were successful.

The early results of impaction grafting are encouraging, and suggest rapid incorporation of the allograft, with reconstitution of the proximal femur (Figure 6.10). Histological analysis of reclaimed specimens confirms the radiological evidence of remodelling. Ling et al.[36] (1993) reports the replacement of allograft chips by viable cortical bone in a femur retrieved 3.5 years after cemented revision with impaction allografting. The cement–tissue interface was similar to that seen after primary arthroplasty. Longer-term results are awaited.

## Infection

The use of modern operating theatres with lami-nar-flow ventilation, antibiotic-impregnated bone cement and prophylactic antibiotics has reduced the incidence of infected joint replacements to only 1–2% of the total. Consequently the typical orthopaedic surgeon will rarely see florid cases of infection. The crucial factor in the treatment of infected arthroplasties is preparation of the environment for reimplantation of a prosthesis.

Confirming the diagnosis may itself be difficult. The diagnosis may be suspected on clinical grounds. A high-grade infection may be obvious with a systemic illness, swinging pyrexia, abscess and sinus formation, etc. This is seldom the case. More often, the typical low-grade infection presents with pain and evidence of prosthetic loosening on plain radiographs. There is a higher incidence of infection following revision surgery — low-grade infections which are overlooked at the time of revision, may in part account for this.

### Preoperative assessment

Prior to undertaking any revision surgery, attempts to exclude active infection are mandatory. Plain radiographs may demonstrate focal lysis or a periosteal reaction. A full blood count (FBC) may

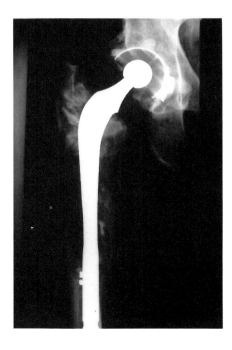

(a)

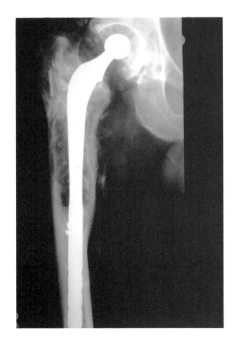

(b)

**Figure 6.10**  Reconstitution of the femur 1 month (a) and 18 months (b) after impaction allografting of an uncemented component.

have a raised neutrophil count and low red cell count, secondary to chronic infection. The erythrocyte sedimentation rate (ESR) and C-reactive protein (CRP) may be elevated. In combination, this is more indicative of infection. Thoren and Wigren[37] studied the ESR in 79 cases of revision surgery and concluded that a sedimentation rate of 35 mm per hour represented an acceptable borderline between infected and non-infected prostheses. However, Roberts et al.[38] include 3 cases of infection with a sedimentation rate below 20 mm per hour.

Increased uptake from $^{99m}$technetium methylenediphosphonate (MDP) bone scan may suggest loosening. Combined with increased uptake from a $^{67}$gallium-citrate (Ga-citrate) scan or a $^{111}$indium-labelled leucocyte scan, the index of suspicion for infection is greater (Figures 6.11 and 6.12). Glithero et al.[39] found isotope-labelled white cell scans to be useful in the diagnosis of infection during the early period after replacement arthroplasty. Sensitivity was insufficient for use as an isolated screening modality.

A positive culture obtained at open surgery is the only sure way to confirm an infection, although cases of false-positive and false-negative cultures arise. The administration of antibiotics preoperatively, or organisms of low virulence, may prevent positive culture results in the microbiology laboratory despite the use of enhanced culture techniques. Where the sensitivities are confirmed, bone cement can be loaded with an appropriate antibiotic, and a high local concentration of antibiotic delivered.

### Preoperative aspiration culture

Preoperative aspiration and culture of an infected arthroplasty remains controversial as results can be disappointing. An accurate positive culture allows more definitive antibiotic treatment if a single stage re-implantation is to be performed. Barrack and Harris[39] recommended preoperative aspiration in selected cases, as they found no patient with a true-positive culture result without clinical and radiographic evidence of infection. There were a high proportion of false-positive results. Gould et al.[41] found no positive aspiration culture results where there was a low index of suspicion, and results were unreliable where the index of suspicion was greater. Roberts et al.[38], are more enthusiastic about preoperative aspiration, using a radiometric culture

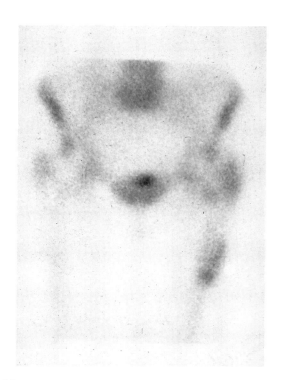

(a)

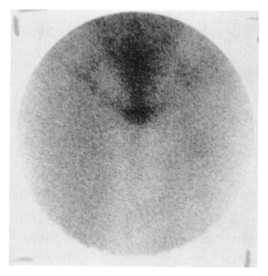

(b)

**Figure 6.11**   a, shows increased uptake from a $^{99m}$Technetium MDP isotope scan; there is no increased uptake of the $^{67}$Ga-citrate isotope scan; b, suggestive of a loose but not infected prosthesis.

technique, reporting 94% correct results with a sensitivity of 87% and 95% specificity.

For aspiration to be of value, extreme care must be exercised during aspiration and the interpretation of enhanced culture results must be with expert assistance of the microbiology department.

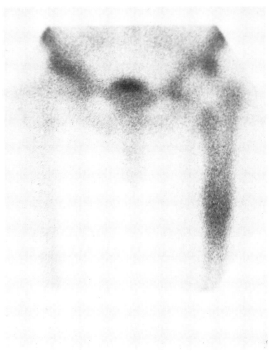

(a)

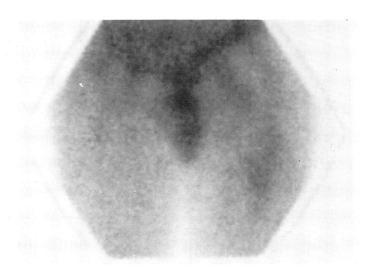

(b)

## Treatment options

The aim of revision surgery in the presence of infection is to eradicate sepsis, maintaining the best possible function. Treatment options (see Table 6.1) include:

- Thorough debridement, followed by continuous lavage
- Excision arthroplasty
- Arthrodesis
- Single-stage exchange (with appropriate bone graft augmentation)
- Two-stage exchange (with appropriate bone graft augmentation).

The results of arthrodesis are poor[42] principally because bone stock may be lost and achieving fusion is difficult; in addition, there may be considerable leg length discrepancy. For young patients, arthrodesis is unacceptable.

## Organisms

The most common organisms identified are the *Staphylococcus epidermidis* and the *Staphylococcus aureus*, although virtually any organism may be identified and occasionally more than one organism is cultured.

## Current practice

The practice of our unit is to undertake a thorough preoperative workup for all revisions, including plain radiographs, FBC, ESR and CRP, $^{99m}$tech-

**Figure 6.12**   In contrast, there is increased uptake from both the $^{99m}$Technetium MDP (a), and the $^{67}$Ga-citrate (b) isotope scans, indicating infection.

netium MDP and [67]Ga-citrate isotope scans. At the time of revision surgery, fluid and tissue are cultured with an enhanced technique in all cases. Where infection is suspected a two-stage revision is undertaken, with a thorough debridement, inserting antibiotic-impregnated cement into the acetabulum and femoral canal at the first stage of revision (Figure 6.13). This is removed at the time of reimplantation, a minimum of three months later. The postoperative culture result is used to administer appropriate antibiotic treatment for the interval before reimplantation and after reimplantation. It is important to ensure peroperative prophylactic antibiotics are not administered until adequate specimens have been obtained.

The undertaking of single-stage revision surgery and augmentation with allograft to restore bone stock, in the presence of infection, is controversial. Morscher et al.[43] advocate a single-stage revision where there is good vasculature, adequate bone stock and a proven organism of low virulence. A success rate of 57% at the first attempt for single-stage revision and a 74% success rate for a two-stage revision is reported. After repeated procedures, for both single- and two-stage revisions, success rates were over 90%. The successful use of allograft is also reported, despite evidence of infection. Berry

et al.[44] report two recurrent infections from a series of 18 patients receiving bone allograft during the second stage of revision for infection. Similarly Loty et al.[45] report good results, with a 9% reinfection rate following single-stage revision, where a high proportion of patients received a bone allograft.

## Excision arthroplasty

Excision of the proximal femur was first popularized by Girdlestone in 1928[46], whose eponym is commonly associated with the procedure, to promote healing after tuberculosis of the hip. Subsequently a Girdlestone excision arthroplasty was advocated as a primary treatment for osteoarthritis of the hip[47]. In current practice, a Girdlestone excision arthroplasty is used principally for the final salvage of a failed replacement arthroplasty, particularly in the presence of deep or resistant infection.

The trend in favour of replacement arthroplasty is ever growing and younger patients are being offered earlier surgery. It is inevitable that revision surgery will be required for younger patients. Likewise, it must be anticipated that in years to come a proportion will be faced with an excision arthroplasty. An appropriately timed excision arthroplasty may save selected patients further extensive and high-risk surgery, with the attendant complications of diminishing leg length and bone stock and possibly the final alternative — amputation.

### Indications

The indications for excision arthroplasty are difficult to define and the final decision rests with the patient and surgeon. Such a decision must be integrated with the patient's age, expectations, previous surgery, volume of residual bone stock, degree of infection, etc, and the alternative options available. Wroblewski[48] proposed the following indications:

1. Inadequate bone stock to secure component fixation using current revision techniques.
2. Repeated surgery in the presence of gross sepsis, scarring, and abductor muscle loss.
3. Extensive soft-tissue infection with mixed or antibiotic-resistant organisms.
4. Patient's general state of health or desire to avoid the possibility or need for further surgery.

Naturally, the extent of the procedure and the patient's anticipated quality of life must be clearly explained.

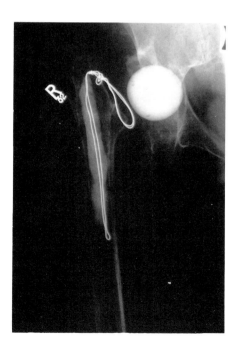

**Figure 6.13** Gentamicin-loaded cement spacers in the acetabulum and femoral canal.

## Surgical technique

This involves the removal of the prosthesis and cement prior to thorough debridement of associated debris. In order to prevent laxity of the hip postoperatively, soft-tissue dissection and bone resection are kept to a minimum. Ideally, the normal anatomy should be left undisturbed. There is a tendency for the limb to adopt a position of external rotation postoperatively. This can be lessened if the psoas tendon is detached from its insertion, transposed around the anterior of the femur and securely reattached to the soft tissues at the posterolateral aspect of the femur. This allows the psoas to act as an internal rotator. The interval between the former acetabulum and the proximal femur should be filled with soft tissue, to obliterate the potential space. This can be achieved by interposing the gluteus medius muscle which should be securely sutured to the soft tissues in the region of the lesser trochanter.

## Postoperative care

In the past, traction has been advocated for a number of weeks prior to mobilization. Manning and Wroblewski[49] found that early mobilization without traction did not affect shortening or wound healing, but reduced the period of hospitalization without prejudice to the final outcome.

There may still be a tendency for the leg to fall into external rotation. This can be corrected with a removable derotation boot, allowing mobilization by day and support whilst in bed.

The requirement for walking aids will reduce as patients regain strength and mobility, and become accustomed to their surgery.

Grauer et al.[50] report a series of 48 Girdlestone resection arthroplasties, 33 were for infection following replacement arthroplasty and the sepsis was eradicated in all but 3 cases. Results were better where the minimum of bone had been resected. Pain was successfully alleviated although the improvement in function was less dramatic, especially in women and following an infected replacement arthroplasty. De Laat et al.[51] reported a good or moderate result in 82.5% of cases from a series of 40 similar cases and Renvall and Einola[52] found a Girdlestone resection arthroplasty to provide an effective functional result when reconstruction was not possible.

## Re-arthroplasty following resection arthroplasty

It is technically feasible in certain circumstances to insert a prosthesis where a previous resection arthroplasty has been performed. Resolution of deep infection is essential and sufficient bone stock is required. Suominen et al.[53] report 20 such cases, with a good result in 15 cases measured as relief of pain and improved hip function. Better results were achieved with a cementless prosthesis in cases of previous infection. Less satisfactory results followed cemented re-arthroplasty and the use of a cementless prosthesis for former aseptic loosening.

# The saddle prosthesis

A saddle prosthesis may be used to provide a stable and mobile articulation between the femur and pelvis, in the presence of advanced bone stock loss and deficient acetabulum (Figure 6.14). In circumstances where the bone stock loss is beyond salvage, this provides a potential solution, without resorting to an excision arthroplasty.

The principle is to provide an extended femoral component, the proximal pole being a saddle-shaped chrome–cobalt surface. The saddle bears directly against the bone of the remaining iliac wing, in place of the deficient acetabulum (Figure 6.15). The prosthesis has also been used for limb salvage and reconstruction following the resection of pelvic bone tumours[54] although massive allograft techniques may now be more appropriate.

## Principle and operative technique

Above a deficient acetabulum the remnant ilium forms a tapered pyramidal shape, with thicker cortical bone on the superomedial surface. This residual robust bone provides the point of articulation.

Surgical dissection must allow adequate exposure of the margins of the ilium above the deficient acetabulum. The soft tissues are stripped, with extreme care to preserve vascular structures, from the medial cortex of the ilium to define the margins of the inner cortex. The apex is fashioned to match the contour of the saddle, allowing for articulation.

A series of adjustments may be made to provide a stable fixation on trial reduction, after appropriate preparation of the femur. To maintain sufficient tension and stability, it is often necessary to over-lengthen the limb by 1–2 cm — there may be some shortening postoperatively. The femoral component is usually secured with pressurized bone cement.

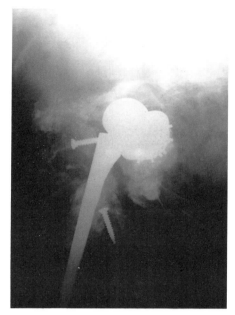

(a)

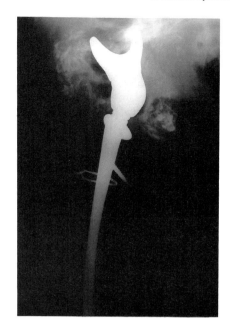

(b)

**Figure 6.14** (a) Advanced bone stock loss in an elderly lady (b) treated with a saddle prosthesis. (Reproduced by kind permission of Mr G.A. Pryor, FRCS, Peterborough, UK.)

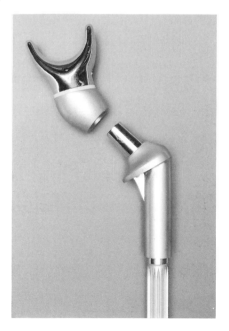

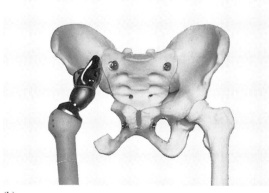

(b)

(a)

**Figure 6.15a,b** The components of the Mark II Waldemar Link Saddle prosthesis (reproduced courtesy of GMBH & Co., Barkhausenweg 10, D-2000, Hamburg 63, Germany).

## Postoperative care

Early mobilization with partial weight-bearing can begin soon after surgery. Patients can then be treated in a manner similar to a conventional primary replacement arthroplasty. There is usually some proximal migration of the prosthesis during early 'bedding-in' of the saddle, combined with radiological sclerosis. Such migration is not seen if the prosthesis is not loaded, but may be greater in the presence of infection.

## Clinical outcome

The saddle prosthesis is used in a limited number of centres as the indications are strictly for the very final stages of limb salvage following revision surgery, and occasionally following massive bone resection. Nieder et al.[55] observed only 76 saddle prostheses were implanted in the course of some 3000 revision procedures at the Endoklinik, and encouraging early results of this series are reported. The clinical outcome in such a variable and endstage group of patients is difficult to evaluate, although the only remaining options are excision arthroplasty or disarticulation.

The early, Mark I, saddle prosthesis has now been replaced by the modified Mark II prosthesis, to allow greater rotation and modularity[56].

## Amputation

Where reconstructive revision surgery has failed, infection proves unremitting, or pain is intolerable, the sole remaining surgical option may be amputation. Amputation will usually be disarticulation through the hip, although a hind-quarter amputation may be required in exceptional circumstances.

Prior to amputation, there may have been extensive surgery with considerable scarring. Achieving good skin closure can be difficult and the advice of a plastic surgeon may be beneficial.

The fitting of a prosthesis, although feasible, may not dramatically improve mobility should the contralateral hip already be diseased.

## References

1. Herberts, P. (1992) Hip arthroplasty revision. *Acta Orthop. Scand.*, **63**, 109–110.
2. Kavanagh, B.F. and Fitzgerald, R.H. (1987) Multiple revisions for failed total hip arthroplasty not associated with infection. *J. Bone Joint Surg.*, **69A** 1144–1149.
3. Repten, J.B., Varmarken, J.E., Sturup, J. et al. (1989) Clinical results after revision and primary hip total arthroplasty. *J. Arthroplasty*, **4**, 297–302.
4. Marti, R.K., Schuller, H.M., Besselaar, P.P. and Vanfrank Haasnoot, E.L. (1990) Results of revision of hip arthroplasty with cement. A five to fourteen year follow-up study. *J. Bone Joint Surg.*, **72A**, 346–354.
5. Retpen, J.B., Varmarken, J.E., Rock, N.D. and Jensen, J.S. (1992) Unsatisfactory results after repeated revision of hip arthroplasty. 61 cases followed for 5 (1–10) years. *Acta Orthop. Scand.*, **63**, 120–127.
6. Dohmae, Y, Bechtold, J.E., Sherman, R.E., et al. (1988). Reduction in cement-bone interface shear strength between primary and revision arthroplasty. *Clin. Orthop.*, **236**, 214–220.
7. Mallory, T.M. (1988) Preparation of the proximal femur in cementless total hip revisions. *Clin. Orthop.*, **235**, 47–60.
8. Lord, G., Marmotte, J.-H., Guillamon, J.-L. and Blanchard, J.-P. (1988) Cementless revision of failed aseptic cemented and cementless total hip arthroplasties: 284 cases. *Clin. Orthop.*, **235**, 67–74.
9. Hedley, A.K., Gruen, T.A. and Ruoff, D.P. (1988) Revision of failed total hip arthroplasties with uncemented porous-coated anatomic components. *Clin. Orthop.*, **235**, 75–90.
10. Engh, C.A., Glassman, A.H., Griffin, W.L. and Mayer, J.G. (1988) Results of cementless revision for failed cemented total hip arthroplasty. *Clin. Orthop.*, **235**, 91–110.
11. McGann, W.A., Welch, R.B. and Picetti, G.D. (1988) Acetabular preparation in cementless revision total hip arthroplasty. *Clin. Orthop.*, **235**, 35–46.
12. Harris, W.H., Krushell, R.J. and Galante, J.O. (1988) Results of cementless revisions of total hip arthroplasties using the Harris–Galante prosthesis. *Clin. Orthop.*, **235**, 120–126.
13. Gustilo, R.B. and Pasternak, H.S. (1988) Revision total hip arthroplasty with titanium ingrowth prosthesis and bone grafting for failed cemented femoral component loosening. *Clin. Orthop.*, **235**, 111–119.
14. Morrey, B.F. and Kavanagh, B.F. (1992) Complications with revision of the femoral component of total hip arthroplasty. Comparison between cemented and uncemented techniques. *J. Arthroplasty*, **7**, 71–79.
15. Padgett, D.E., Kull, L., Rosenburg, A. et al. (1993) Revision of the acetabular component without cement after total hip arthroplasty. *J. Bone Joint Surg.*, **75A**, 663–673.
16. Archibald, D.A.A., Protheroe, K., Stother, I.G. and Campbell, A. (1988) A simple technique for acetabular revision: brief report. *J. Bone Joint Surg.*, **70B**, 838.
17. McMinn, D.J.W., Roberts, P. and Forward, G.R. (1991) A new approach to the hip for revision surgery. *J. Bone Joint Surg.*, **73B**, 899–901.
18. Grigoris P, Roberts, P., McMinn, D.J.W. and Villar, R.N. (1993) A technique for removing an intrapelvic acetabular cup. *J. Bone Joint Surg.*, **75B**, 25–27.
19. D'Antonio, J.A., Capello, W.N., Borden, L.S. et al. (1989) Classification and management of acetabular abnormalities in total hip arthroplasty. *Clin. Orthop.*, **243**, 126–137.
20. Berry, D.J. and Müller, M.E. (1992) Revision arthroplasty using an antiprotrusio cage for massive acetabular bone deficiency. *J. Bone Joint Surg.*, **74B**, 711–715.
21. Rosson, J. and Schatzker, J. (1992) The use of reinforcement rings to reconstruct deficient acetabula. *J. Bone Joint Surg.*, **74B**, 716–720.
22. McMinn, D.J.W. (1993) The ring principle. *J. Bone Joint Surg.*, **75B**, S48.

23. Englebrecht, D.J., Weber, F.A., Sweet, M.B.E. and Jakim, I. (1990) Long term results of revision total hip arthroplasty. *J. Bone Joint Surg.*, **72B**, 41–45.

24. Kershaw, C.J., Atkins, R.M., Dodd, C.A.F. and Bulstrode, C.J.K. (1991) Revison total hip arthroplasty for aseptic failure. *J. Bone Joint Surg.*, **73B**, 564–568.

25. Strömberg, C.N., Herberts, P. and Palmertz, B. (1992) Cemented revision hip arthroplasty. A multicenter 5–9 year study of 204 first revisions for loosening. *Acta Orthop. Scand.*, **63**, 111–119.

26. Pellici, P.M., Wilson, P.D., Sledge, C.B. et al. (1985) Long term results of revision total hip replacement. *J. Bone Joint Surg.*, **67A**, 513–516.

27. Emerson, R.H., Malinin, T.I., Cuellar, A.D. et al. (1992) Cortical strut allografts in the reconstruction of the femur in revision total hip arthroplasty. A basic science and clinical study. *Clin. Orthop.*, **285**, 35–44.

28. Chandler, H.P. and Penenberg, B.L. (1989) Femoral reconstruction. In *Bone Deficiency in Total Hip Replacements* (H.P. Chandler and B.L. Penenberg, eds.) Thorofare, New Jersey: Slack, p. 116.

29. Rodrigio, J.J., Martin, R.B., Reynolds, H.B. et al. (1990) Interlocking femoral components for revision arthroplasty with allografts. *J. Arthroplasty*, **5**, S35–41.

30. Allan, D.G., Lavoie, G.J., McDonald, S. et al. (1991) Proximal femoral allografts in revision hip arthroplasty. *J. Bone Joint Surg.*, **73B**, 235–240.

31. McDermott, A.G.P., Langer, F., Pritzker, K.P.H. and Gross, A.E. (1985) Fresh small fragment osteochondral allografts: long term follow-up study on the first 100 cases. *Clin. Orthop.*, **197**, 96–102.

32. Simon, J.P., Fowler, J.L., Gie, G.A. et al. (1991) Impaction cancellous grafting of the femur in cemented total hip revision arthroplasty. *J. Bone Joint Surg.*, **73B**, S73.

33. Gie, G.A., Linder, L., Ling, R.S,M., et al. (1993) Impacted cancellous autograft and cement for revision total hip arthroplasty. *J. Bone Joint Surg.*, **75B**, 14–21.

34. Sloof, T.J.J.H., Huiskes, R., van Horn, J. and Lemmens, A.J. (1984) Bone grafting in total hip replacement for acetabular protrusion. *Acta Orthop. Scand.*, **55**, 593–596.

35. Nelson, I.W., Bulstrode, C.J.K. and Mowat, A.G. (1990) Femoral allografts in revision of hip replacement. *J. Bone Joint Surg.*, **72B**, 151–152.

36. Ling, R.S.M., Timperley, A.J. and Linder, L. (1993) Histology of cancellous impaction grafting in the femur. *J. Bone Joint Surg.*, **75B** 693–696.

37. Thoren, B. and Wigren, A. (1991) Erythrocyte sedimentation rate in infection of total hip replacements. *Orthopaedics*, **14**, 495–497.

38. Roberts, P., Walters, A.J. and McMinn, D.J.W. (1992) Diagnosing infection in hip replacements. *J. Bone Joint Surg.*, **74B**, 265–269.

39. Glithero, P.R., Grigoris, P., Harding, L.K. et al. (1993) White cell scans and infected joint replacements. *J. Bone Joint Surg.*, **75B**, 371–374.

40. Barrack, R.L. and Harris, W.H. (1993) The value of aspiration of the hip joint before revision total hip arthroplasty. *J. Bone Joint Surg.*, **75A**, 66–76.

41. Gould, E.S., Potter, H.G. and Bober, S.E. (1990) Role of routine percutaneous hip aspirations prior to prosthesis revision. *Skeletal Radiology*, **19**, 427–430.

42. McDonald, D.J., Fitzgerald, R.H. and Ilstrup, D.M. (1989) Two-stage reconstruction of a total hip arthroplasty because of infection. *J. Bone Joint Surg.*, **71A**, 828–834.

43. Morscher, E., Babst, R. and Jenny, H. (1990) Treatment of infected joint arthroplasty. *Int. Orthop.*, **14** 161–165.

44. Berry, D.J., Chandler, H.P. and Reilly, D.T. (1991) The use of bone grafts in two-stage reconstruction after failure of hip replacements due to infection. *J. Bone Joint Surg.*, **73A**, 1460–1468.

45. Loty, B., Postel, M., Evrard, J. et al. (1992) One stage revision of infected total hip replacements with replacement of the bone loss by allografts. Study of 90 cases of which 46 used bone allografts. *Int. Orthop.*, **16**, 330–338.

46. Girdlestone, G.R. (1928) Arthrodesis and other operations for tuberculosis of the hip. *The Robert Jones Birthday Volume*, London: Oxford University Press, p. 134.

47. Taylor, R.G. (1950) Pseudoarthrosis of the hip joint. *J. Bone Joint Surg.*, **32B**, 161–165.

48. Wroblewski, B.M. (1984) Girdlestone pseudarthrosis following deep sepsis in total hip arthroplasty. In: N.S. Eftekhar (ed) *Infection in Joint Replacement. Prevention and Management*, St Louis: Mosby, pp. 345–362.

49. Manning, M.P. and Wroblewski, B.M. (1993) Girdlestone pseudarthrosis following hip replacement. Is traction necessary? *J. Bone Joint Surg.*, **75B**, S40.

50. Grauer, J.D., Amstutz, H.C., O'Carroll, P.F. and Dorey, F.J. (1989) Resection arthroplasty of the hip. *J. Bone Joint Surg.*, **71A**, 669–678.

51. De Laat, E.A., van der List, J.J., van Horn, J.R. and Sloof, T.J. (1991) Girdlestone's pseudarthrosis after removal of a total hip prosthesis; a retrospective study of 40 patients. *Acta Orthop. Belgica*, **57**, 109–113.

52. Renvall, S. and Einola, S. (1990) Girdlestone operation. An acceptable alternative in the case of unreconstructable hip arthroplasty. *Annales Chirurgiae et Gynaecologiae*, **79**, 165–167.

53. Suominen, S., Ragni, P., Lindholm, S. and Antti-Poika, I. (1990) A comparison between cemented and cementless implants in revision arthroplasty of the hip following resection arthroplasty. *Ital. J. Orthop. Trauma*, **16**, 159–167.

54. Van der Lei, B., Hoekstra, H.J., Veth, R.P. et al. (1992) The use of the saddle prosthesis for reconstruction of the hip joint after tumour resection of the pelvis. *J. Surg. Oncology*, **50**, 216–219.

55. Nieder, E., Elson, R.A., Engelbrecht, E. et al. (1990) The saddle prosthesis for salvage of the destroyed acetabulum. *J. Bone Joint Surg.*, **72B**, 1014–1022.

56. Nieder, E. and Keller, A. (1989) The saddle prosthesis Mark II, Endo-Modell. In *New Developments for Limb Salvage in Musculoskeletal Tumours*, T. Yamamuro, ed. Tokyo: Springer-Verlag, pp. 481–490.

# 7

# Surgical approaches and instrumentation

Thomas H. Mallory, Maria B. Mitchell and Robert W. Eberle

## Introduction

The challenge of performing revision total hip replacement (THR) is quite formidable and brings forth many technical complexities. Mastering a versatile exposure technique will provide a suitable environment for optimum cement removal and stabilization of the soft-tissue envelope. Femoral cement removal can be precarious as debonding of the cement mantle from the bony interface is seldom complete and is further complicated by the extrusion of the cement mantle into the distal medullary canal. Acetabular cement removal is equally difficult due to the intrusion of cement into the recesses of the acetabular cavity. Competency in the technical aspects of revision total hip replacement saves the surgeon precious operative time, anxiety, fatigue, and minimizes injury to the host tissues. Therefore, the orthopaedic surgeon performing revision THR must select a surgical approach and method or methodologies of cement removal which are direct, efficient, and safe.

## Surgical exposure

The goals of surgical exposure in THR should include visualization of the proximal femur and the acetabulum without compromise to the neurovascular or bony structures in and about the hip. The exposure should maintain an adequate soft-tissue envelope for revascularization of an area which has become ischaemic and possibly debris-laden while the lengthy, complex reconstruction is being performed.

Although there have been many surgical approaches developed and advocated for primary and revision THR, all have intrinsic advantages and disadvantages[1–5]. Many surgeons prefer the posterior approach as it preserves the abductor muscle cuff and affords easy accessibility to the hip joint. The disadvantage to this approach is the potential for instability and subsequent dislocation as well as sciatic nerve compromise. Especially in revision THR, the transtrochanteric approach allows excellent exposure to both the proximal femur and the acetabulum. However, if the trochanter does not heal completely, abductor function can be lost, resulting in limp and instability. The trochanteric slide approach is based on maintaining the integrity of the abductor-trochanter-vastus lateralis muscle complex. The anatomical continuity is accomplished by creating a thin fragment of trochanter which, in turn, allows preservation of this complex muscle cuff. Once the trochanter fragment or *wafer* has been created, the entire muscle complex can be slid anterior or posterior, depending on the surgeon's preference. At the completion of the operation, reattachment of the trochanteric fragment is still necessary and not always easily accomplished. Once again, if the trochanteric fragment fails to unite, muscle instability and/or painful bursitis may persist.

The anterolateral approach offers the surgeon versatility of entry into the hip joint[6–8]. The incision can be easily extended caudad or cephalad for maximum visualization of the femoral shaft or acetabulum, while avoiding osteotomy of the greater trochanter and preserving the muscle cuff. The approach maintains a continuous musculo-tendinous envelope which restores active abductor function, maintains stability and affords gait normalcy. There are three variations of the anterolateral approach that address the various aspects of revision THR.

## Anterolateral exposure technique

### Type I

The Type I anterolateral exposure is an approach that provides limited regional access to the acetabulum and proximal femur (Figure 7.1). With the patient placed in the full lateral decubitus position, the skin incision is extended from the greater trochanter cephalad in a straight direction to the level of the iliac spine. The incision extends caudal along the midshaft of the femur approximately 8 cm. The skin and subcutaneous tissues are divided in the direction of the incision. The muscle fibres of the gluteus maximus are split superiorly exposing the muscle mass of the gluteus minimus-medius complex. The surgeon inserts a finger beneath the anterior border of the abductor muscle mass to identify the position of the prosthetic device (Figure 7.2). The location of the prosthetic device references the point at which a longitudinal split is made in the abductor muscle mass. The muscle split is extended anteriorly and superiorly following the direction of the abductor muscle fibres. The proximal anterior-superior extent of the muscle split courses approximately 1 cm above the superior border of the acetabulum. The muscle division continues distally along the anterior border of the greater trochanter, then moves posteriorly beneath the vastus lateralis ridge coursing distal along the linea aspera to the level of the insertion of the gluteus maximus tendon. Following the completion of the muscle split, a partial capsulectomy is performed to expose the joint. The surgeon dislocates the femoral component anteriorly. Release of the iliopsoas muscle and posterior capsule structures allows further mobilization of the femur. While working with the femur, the involved extremity is maintained in a flexed, adducted and externally-rotated position. To enhance acetabular exposure, the involved

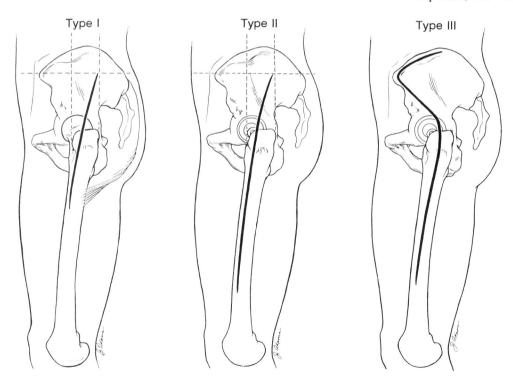

**Figure 7.1**   Three variations of the anterolateral exposure; Type I: An exposure suitable for index arthroplasty or limited revision hip replacement, Type II: Distal extension of exposure to facilitate prosthetic extraction and reconstructive procedures of the bone-defecit femur, Type III: Extensile exposure offers complete access and visualization of the acetabulum and femur while preserving neurovascular structures to the gluteus minimus and medius.

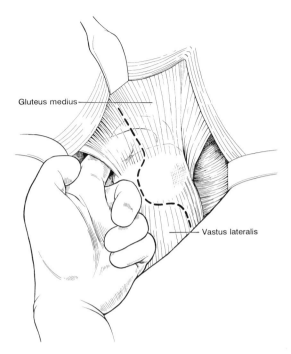

Gluteus medius

Vastus lateralis

**Figure 7.2**   Palpation of the prosthetic device identifies the location of the longitudinal abductor muscle split.

extremity is extended and positioned posterior to the acetabulum. Acetabular exposure is further enhanced with the appropriate placement of retractors in the four quadrants of the acetabular region.

Following completion of the reconstructive procedure, appropriate tension within the abductor muscle is determined by measuring leg length equality against the contralateral extremity. The abductor muscle mass is tensed by the lateral offset of the femoral prosthetic component. The abductor muscle split, or separation, is repaired by approximation of the muscle sleeve to its original position along the anterolateral surface of the femur with a heavy, #5, non-absorbable suture. The limited anterolateral exposure is recommended when the dimensions of the revision operation, including prosthetic extraction and reimplantation, require a working field similar to that of an index operation.

## Type II

This modified anterolateral exposure is proposed for situations in which acetabular reconstruction is neither complex nor involved, but requires extensile femoral exposure which will facilitate not only

prosthetic extraction but reconstitution of deficient bony structures. The skin incision is merely a distal or caudal extension of approach Type I (see Figure 7.1). This modification is determined by the necessity of the lateral thigh exposure required for prosthetic extraction manoeuvres as well as reconstitution of the proximal and mid-femoral shaft. The exposure moves distal across the lateral muscle planes, separating the vastus lateralis along the linea aspera femoris. The muscle mass of the quadriceps is moved anteriorly, exposing the lateral and anterior portions of the femur. The muscle envelope continues proximally, extending into the anterior fibres of the abductor muscle mass. The lateral abductor muscle fibres of the gluteus medius remain attached to the posterior border of the greater trochanter. It is necessary to release the iliopsoas muscle and to skeletonize the posterior capsule from the proximal femur to facilitate exposure. With this exposure, the muscle envelope including the quadriceps muscle-abductor complex remains intact and, although separated from osseous structures, maintains a continuous soft-tissue muscle cuff. This approach allows excellent exposure of the proximal femur for removal of prosthetic femoral components and cement and for any type of subsequent bone grafting procedures to reconstitute the osseous structures. It affords excellent visualization, which can serve to monitor the extraction processes while identifying perforations or areas of bony discontinuity in the femur.

Following reconstitution of the proximal femur and prosthetic reimplantation, the muscle tension in the abductor-quadriceps muscle complex is determined by the lateral displacement of the shaft of the femur which, again, is facilitated by the offset of the prosthetic component utilized. The abductor-quadriceps complex is reattached to the lateral border of the femur by securing it at various points with heavy, #5, non-absorbable suture.

## Type III

This extensile exposure involves the development of the revision anterolateral incision cephalad to enhance the exposure of the acetabulum while preserving the integrity of the neurovascular structures supplying the gluteus minimus and medius (Figure 7.1). The neurovascular structures enter from the sciatic notch and pass anteriorly 4–5 cm above the lateral edge of the acetabulum. In order to maintain the integrity of the neurovascular structures, the anterolateral approach must extend toward the

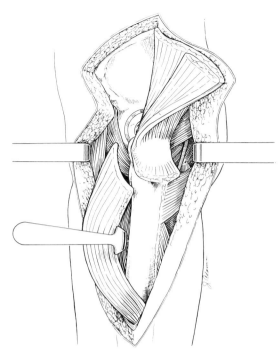

**Figure 7.3** Subperiosteal elevation of the abductor mass off the wing of the ilium exposes the anterior, posterior and superior regions of the acetabulum.

anterior superior iliac spine and then course cephalad and posteriorly along the crest of the ilium. The abductor muscle mass is elevated subperiosteally from the wing of the ilium (Figure 7.3). This approach offers excellent exposure to the anterior, superior and posterior regions of the acetabulum.

Through this extensile incision it is also possible to enter the inner pelvic table by developing an expanded interval between the iliacus muscle which lays against the inner pelvic wing of the ilium. With blunt dissection, the iliacus muscle is lifted off the inner pelvic table and a limited, but effective, entry point is created for removal of intrapelvic cement, screws or other elements that may have penetrated the medial wall of the acetabulum. Also, it is possible to identify and avoid the neurovascular bundle which is located anterior and medial to the iliacus muscle.

Following reconstruction of the acetabulum, the abductor muscle mass is secured to the wing of the ilium by attachment to the abdominal fascia. By combining approaches Type II and Type III, the entire lateral aspects of the pelvis, as well as the

proximal and mid portions of the femur can be exposed for any revision THR situation. These incisions follow muscle planes and are essentially muscle-splitting dissections, rather than transverse resection of muscle mass and bone. Therefore, exposure and wound closure are easily performed with minimal disruption to the soft-tissue envelope about the hip joint.

# Cement removal in total hip replacement

The objective is to remove the prosthesis efficiently, together with the cement mantle, while maximally preserving the surrounding osseous structure. The accomplishment of these objectives requires preoperative planning, special instrumentation, and visual conceptualization of the reconstruction arthroplasty.

# Preoperative planning

Planning for a revision THR operation includes a critical serial radiographic analysis evaluating the prosthetic type, progression of bone destruction, the location and amount of bone cement to be removed, and the anticipated bone profile of what will remain for reconstruction of the prosthetic composite. An appropriate X-ray must be available for full visualization during a revision THR, thus providing the surgeon a road map to direct the course of the operative procedure.

The cement removal instrumentation needed to execute a successful revision THR can vary from sharp, angulated osteotomes to high-speed, power-driven burrs and drills. Recently, the introduction of ultrasonic, high-frequency instrumentation has facilitated cement removal.[9,10] Additional equipment, including special retractors which enhance exposure and devices which assist in the extraction of the prosthetic composite, is helpful. It is important that an effective ingress-egress fluid system and suction devices are readily available for the removal of accumulated fluids and debris produced during the procedure.

# Removal of the cemented acetabular component

Familiarity with bony landmarks is imperative in identification of the osseous structures of the

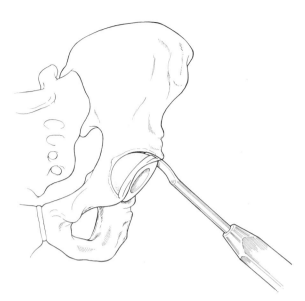

**Figure 7.4**   A series of curved osteotomes are used to violate the prosthetic-cement interface.

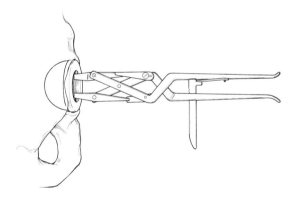

**Figure 7.5**   A cup extraction instrument captures the acetabular component from an inside-outside dimension for ease of removal.

acetabulum. Superiorly, the gluteal muscle mass must be lifted from the lateral edge of the acetabulum. In the removal of a cemented acetabular component, the interface between the prosthesis and the cement must be debonded. Breaking the prosthetic–cement interface is recommended regardless of whether the component is metal-backed or all polyethylene. This is accomplished by using of a series of curved osteotomes inserted into the prosthetic–cement interface (Figure 7.4).

By entering at the prosthetic–cement interface, the polymethylmethacrylate (PMMA) serves as a protector for the acetabular bone stock. The interface is broken circumferentially along the contour of the acetabular component while carefully maintaining the integrity of the cement thereby protecting the adjacent bony structures. Ultrasonic, high-frequency driven instrumentation can facilitate the debonding process by vibrating curved acetabular osteotomes through the prosthetic–cement interface. Once the cup is broken free from the cement mantle, the component is removed from the cement bed. Acetabular component extraction can be performed by gripping the edge of the component with a sharp instrument or by levering the cup out with cup extractor instrumentation. The extraction instrumentation captures the acetabular component from an inside-out dimension creating a long, lever-arm extraction force thus easing component removal (Figure 7.5).

## Acetabular cement removal

PMMA is a brittle material and can be fragmented into cleavage planes by striking the cement mass with sharp instruments. The cement fragments are then easily removed from the osseous bed. In the process of acetabular cement removal, it is important that the periphery of the acetabulum be exposed and the interface between the cement and the bone be clearly identified. It is important not to penetrate too deeply into the cement–bone interface while attempting to lever the instruments against the bony bed. By levering against the bone, there is an increased risk of breaking the peripheral acetabular bony ring which can make reconstitution of the acetabulum difficult. Therefore, one must debond or break the interface about the periphery by moving the osteotomes toward the centre of the acetabulum thereby levering the cement inwardly while avoiding contact with the peripheral bony ring of the acetabulum. Once the peripheral cement has been broken and removed, one is left with a central cement mass which often adheres to the dome of the acetabulum. This region of cement is best removed by creating a series of vertical and longitudinal cracks across the cement by simply striking the cement with a sharp osteotome. Once the cement is fragmented, it is easily removed from the floor of the acetabulum. When removing acetabular cement, preoperative AP and lateral X-rays must be visible to the operating surgeon. Frequent reference to the AP X-ray gives the surgeon the profile of the cement and allows one to determine where the cement mass is located. Often there is a question as to how much cement actually needs to be removed in order to create a successful reconstruction. If there is no sepsis, the amount of cement needed to be removed strictly involves the peripheral ring and the dome of the acetabulum. In most cases intrapelvic cement should be left alone. If there is a large amount of intrapelvic cement that needs to be removed, the anterior pillar of the acetabulum should be exposed and the iliacus muscle lifted from the pelvic floor. The surgeon places his hand under the iliacus muscle, into the intrapelvic space, and identifies the cement mass and then simply pushes it through the bony aperture. This point of entry into the intrapelvic region is safe and avoids the danger of creating haemorrhage. It is imperative that no sharp instruments be used to explore the intrapelvic region. The surgeon's hand alone can be used as a safe and effective tool for performing this blunt dissection.

## Removal of a cemented femoral component

Removal of a cemented component from the proximal femur is facilitated by creating a large step cut, in the shape of an 'L', at the level of the lesser trochanter, beneath the component collar, at the junction of the neck of the prosthetic device. It is important that this region is clear of soft tissue, bone, cement, and debris to aid the debonding and extraction processes. The prosthetic device is then driven retrograde from the proximal femur. The lateral region must be clear of any obstruction as it may create significant blockage and subsequent fracture of the greater trochanter.

Early designed, cemented femoral components are easily extracted by the use of a mallet and a blunt driver. Sharp blows against the prosthetic component disengages the device from the cement mantle. In cases of a collarless, cemented prosthesis, a sharp-tipped, hardened punch can be used to drive the prosthesis retrograde. A locking wrench device may be used to grip the femoral neck of the prosthesis and, with the use of a slap hammer, disengagement of the prosthetic device from the cement mantle can be accomplished. In the case of modular prostheses, the removal of the modular head leaves the neck of the prosthesis exposed. The Bohn extractor (Biomet Inc., Warsaw, Indiana), a locking wrench type device, can be used to grip the

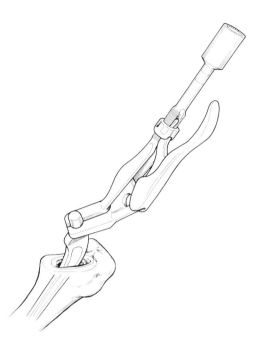

**Figure 7.6** The Bohn Extractor (Biomet, Inc., Warsaw, IN), a locking-wrench device, is used to grip the neck of the femoral component, and, in conjunction with a slap-hammer, facilitates disengagement of the prosthetic device from the cement mantle.

neck of the prosthesis for extraction (Figure 7.6). In extracting cemented femoral components, a retrograde force is more efficient than trying to extract the device with an 'in-and-out' toggle force applied at the head–neck junction. If extraction of the prosthetic device proves difficult, further removal of the cement mantle in the upper one-third of the femur may be required.

The most difficult types of cemented prostheses to remove are those devices in which an attempt is made to enhance the bond between the cement and the prosthesis. Characteristically, these prostheses are precoated with methylmethacrylate or manufactured with a textured surface. With the use of femoral apertures such as windows, gutters or troughs, the insertion of fine, thin, pencil-shaped, pneumatic-driven drills can aid in debonding the bone–cement and cement–component interfaces[11,12]. If the prosthetic interface between the cement and the metal is not broken, attempts to extract the device can create severe bone deficits or fracture of the proximal femur that may contribute to the failure of the reconstructive composite.

## Removing cement from the femoral canal

When removing cement from the femoral canal, it is important to understand that there are three distinct regions of the femur that are occupied by the cement mantle. Zone 1 is the region from the lesser trochanter proximally. Zone 2 from is the lesser trochanter distally through the region of the isthmus approximately 10 cm. Zone 3 is distal to the isthmus and is the region where cement occupies the femoral canal distal to the prosthetic profile.

### Zone 1

Removal of cement from Zone 1 is easily accomplished with the use of sharp osteotomes which create cleavage planes in the cement (Figure 7.7).

The cement mantle is then easily fragmented and removed. When entering the bone–cement interface, the surgeon must lever the osteotome towards the centre of the bone and not against the lateral bony periphery, thereby avoiding fracture of the proximal bone envelope.

### Zone 2

Zone 2 is often a difficult area from which to remove the cement. Due to the narrowing and curving internal dimensions of the femur in the region of the isthmus, direct visualization is impaired. Often, the bone has been weakened by the generation of particulate debris and the resultant osteolytic process. The technique of controlled perforation is used to attain direct visualization of the cement mantle in the mid and distal femur

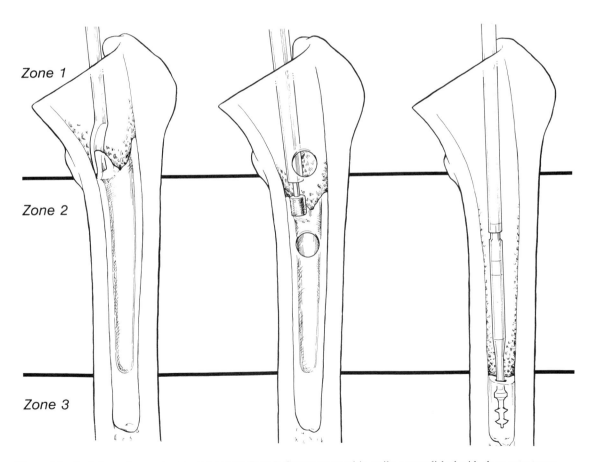

**Figure 7.7** Technique of cement removal by zone; Zone I: Cement removal is easily accomplished with sharp osteotomes, Zone II: The technique of controlled perforation is used to attain direct visualization while removing the cement mantle in the mid and distal femur, Zone III: Ultrasonic instruments melt the cement mantle while avoiding perforation of the distal tube.

(Figure 7.7). Controlled perforation is accomplished by lifting the quadriceps muscle off the anterior shaft of the femur and then making a series of oval apertures in the anterior cortex of the bone with the use of a high-speed drill. The minimum spacing of each anterior aperture is two times the diameter of the femur. By directing the reamer along the course of the bony apertures, the surgeon can follow, under direct vision, the position of the reamer at all times. The cement is quickly removed from this region of the femoral canal with decreased risk of inadvertent perforation of the bone. An additional advantage of controlled perforations is the ingress and egress of irrigation fluids through the apertures. Light can also enter the canal through these openings and greatly increases the visualization capacity. The perforation apertures heal rapidly and need no further attention[13,14].

## Zone 3

Removal of bone cement from Zone 3 can be the most challenging. Recently, with the introduction of ultrasonic, high-frequency instrumentation, cement removal from this region has been greatly enhanced[10]. The ultrasonic instruments melt the cement mantle while avoiding perforation of the bony tube (Figure 7.7). In addition, these instruments can be used blindly by pushing the vibrating tip against the cement while moving it distally as the cement melts. A high-pitched noise is created when the instrument butts against the bone, however, there is silence when the instrument is vibrating against the cement. The tactile sensitivity is quite keen and the surgeon quickly learns to differentiate between instrumentation placed against the cement versus bone.

Alternative methods of removal of cement from Zone 3 are fraught with increased complexities and risks[11,15–21]. Although controlled perforations can be made in Zone 3, it is difficult to direct the course of the reamer along the curvature of the femoral canal. One is more likely to inadvertently perforate the bone even though direct visualization of the straight pneumatic reamers is possible. Under the most extreme conditions, it is recommended that a transverse osteotomy of the distal third of the femur be performed just beyond the physiological curve of the femur. This manoeuvre allows access to the distal femoral composite and, therefore, facilitates the insertion of straight reamers into the distal fragment for complete removal of the cement mantle. After an osteotomy has been made, the use of fracture plates or onlay cortical

strut grafts are recommended when reconstructing Zone 3.

It is important for the surgeon to understand that in cement removal, exposure and opening of the medullary canal may seem radical but, in the long run, is conservative. The bony apertures heal, the windows can be closed with onlay cortical strut grafts and the bony tube maintained in areas of compression and tension[8]. Creation of an aperture for visualization within the bony tube of the femur along the anterior cortex is recommended rather than trying to remove cement blindly with instruments that can cause inadvertent fractures and significantly weaken the bone construct. As more and more revision surgeries become necessary, it is important to develop a system of cement removal which is quick and efficient without running the risk of damaging the bony envelope.

## Conclusions

Simplicity, efficiency and safety are essential ingredients in the surgical exposure and cement removal in revision THR. The anterolateral surgical exposure is versatile and allows an expansion of the incision to incorporate all complexities of total joint replacement including extensive exposures of the acetabular and femoral regions. It maintains muscle planes, it allows for rapid reconstitution of muscle function and leaves an environment for revascularization of muscle and osseous structures.

Acetabular component removal is generally easy and involves the debonding of the prosthetic composite from the cement and a simple levering of the device free from the cement cavity. Cement removed from the acetabulum is debonded peripherally and then fractured, fragmented and extracted from the acetabular dome. Intrapelvic cement should only be removed when there is impingement or obstruction to vital organs or when there is a history of sepsis.

Proximal femoral component removal is enhanced by creating a large L-cut beneath the prosthetic composite and removing the device in a retrograde fashion. Special circumstances involve prosthetic systems in which there has been an attempt to bond the prosthetic device to the cement mantle. In cases of this type, adequate exposure and an attempt to debond or break the interface within the composite facilitates extraction. Cement removal from the proximal femur is simplified when one understands the regional differences that are represented by the bone anatomy. Zones 1, 2 and 3 refer to a proximal-to-distal classification of the femur. Cement in Zone 1 is easily removed by sharp instruments that fragment and break the cement. Zone 2 is the region of the internal contour of the femur where limited visualization of the prosthetic composite exists. Cement removal from this area is enhanced with the use of controlled perforation. Zone 3 is a challenging and difficult region of the femur to remove cement. The recent introduction of ultrasonic technology has improved this dangerous task. It is occasionally necessary to osteotomize the femur in Zone 3 to completely remove the cement should it be necessary.

By following these techniques for preoperative planning, surgical exposure and prosthetic composite removal for revision THR, the surgeon saves precious operative time, anxiety, fatigue, and minimizes injury to the host tissues thus providing the patient with an optimum revision milieu.

# References

1. Dall, D. (1986) Exposure of the hip by anterior osteotomy of the greater trochanter: A modified anterolateral approach. *J. Bone Joint Surg.*, **68B**, 382–386.
2. Foster, D. and Hunter, J.R. (1987) The direct lateral approach to the hip for arthroplasty: Advantages and complications. *Orthopaedics*, **10**, 274–280.
3. Gibson, A. (1950) Posterior exposure of the hip joint. *J. Bone Joint Surg.*, **32B**, 183–186.
4. Hardinge, K. (1982) The direct lateral approach to the hip. *J. Bone Joint Surg.*, **64B**, 17–19.
5. Stephenson, P.K. and Freeman, M.A.R. (1991) Exposure of the hip using a modified anterolateral approach. *J. Arthroplasty*, **6**, 137–150.
6. Head, W.C., Mallory, T.H., Berklacich, F.M. et al. (1987) Extensile exposure of the hip for revision arthroplasty. *J. Arthroplasty*, **2**, 265–274.
7. Mallory, T.H. (1992) Surgical exposure and cement removal in revision total hip arthroplasty. *Semin. Arthroplasty*, **3(4)**, 257–263.
8. Lombardi, A.V. Jr (1992) Cement removal in revision total hip arthroplasty. *Semin. Arthroplasty*, **3(4)**, 264–272.
9. Caillouette, J.T., Gorab, R.S., Klapper, R.C. and Anzel, S.H. (1991) Revision arthroplasty facilitated by ultrasonic tool cement removal. Part I: in vitro evaluation. *Orthop. Rev.*, **20**, 353–357.
10. Caillouette, J.T., Gorab R.S., Klapper, R.C. and Anzel, S.H. (1991) Revision arthroplasty facilitated by ultrasonic tool cement removal. Part II: Histological analysis of endosteal bone after cement removal. *Orthop. Rev.*, **20**, 435–440.
11. Moreland, J.R., Marder, R. and Anspach, W.E. Jr (1986) The window technique for the removal of broken femoral stems in total hip replacement. *Clin. Orthop.*, **212**, 245–249.
12. Moreland, J.R. (1991) Techniques for removal of the prosthesis and cement in hip revisional arthroplasty. In *Advances in Total Hip Reconstruction* (H. Tullos, ed.). Instructional Course Lectures. Park Ridge, Il, American Academy of Orthopaedic Surgery, vol. 40, pp. 163–170.
13. Dennis, D.A., Dingman, C.A., Meglan, D.A. et al. (1987) Femoral cement removal in revision total hip arthroplasty: A biomechanical analysis. *Clin. Orthop.*, **220**, 142–147.
14. Sydney, S.V. and Mallory, T.H. (1990) Controlled perforation. A safe method of cement removal from the femoral canal. *Clin. Orthop.*, **253**, 168–171.
15. Muller, M.E. (1970) Total hip prosthesis. *Clin. Orthop.*, **72**, 46–68.
16. Cameron, H.U. (1990) Femoral windows for easy cement removal in hip revision surgery. *Orthop. Rev.*, **19**, 909–912.
17. Nelson, C.L. and Weber, M.J. (1981) Technique in windowing the femoral shaft for removal of bone cement. *Clin. Orthop.*, **154**, 336–337.
18. Nelson, C.L. and Barnes, C.L. (1990) Removal of bone cement from the femoral shaft using a femoral windowing device. *J. Arthroplasty*, **5**, 67–69.
19. Turner, T.H. and Emerson, R.H. Jr (1982) Femoral revision total hip arthroplasty. In *Revision Total Hip Arthroplasty* (R.H. Turner and A.D. Scheller Jr, eds) New York, Grune & Stratton, pp. 75–106.
20. Razzano, C.D. (1977) Removal of methylmethacrylate in failed total hip arthroplasties: An improved technique. *Clin. Orthop.*, **126**, 181–182.
21. Eftekhar, N.S. (1977) Rechannelization of cemented femur using a guide and drill system. *Clin. Orthop.*, **123**, 29–31.

# 8

# Femoral impaction allografting

Richard N. Villar

## Introduction

Though the use of allograft bone is not new, the past decade has demonstrated an explosion in its use within orthopaedic surgery. This has been largely brought about by the rising numbers of complex revision procedures undertaken by many orthopaedic centres, even though the use of allograft tissue is applicable to many different aspects of orthopaedic surgery.

During femoral reconstruction, allograft bone may be used in a variety of forms: massive or morsellized, frozen or freeze-dried, strut or corticocancellous, and so on. There is no one variety of allograft that is suitable for all situations, so it is wise that the surgeon has a broad range of tissues available if revision surgery is planned. For many operations, a combination of allograft designs will be needed, a common mixture being morsellized and strut ('patch') allograft. But whatever variety is chosen, the principle remains the same. Allograft needs to be fixed tight to the recipient, or impacted tight. Loose application of allograft bone may be asking for trouble.

It is now realized that one should not ignore the problem of reduced bone stock at revision surgery. Multiple revision procedures are now the norm for many patients, and can only approach success if the bone at the operation site is of reasonable quality. Traditionally, recementation has been used, but this can be associated with high levels of failure[1,2], particularly so if bone stock is deficient. Results are equally unsatisfactory after repeated revisions[3]. Not all are pessimistic about the use of cemented revision procedures[4], particularly when modern cementing techniques are used[5].

At operation, it is common to find a ballooned, thin, smooth, ivory-like surface to the inner femoral cortex. When faced with this situation it is not surprising that cementation to such a surface has such weak shear strength[6]. Somehow that weakened surface must be strengthened — impaction grafting is one good, widely-used, alternative.

In theory, the technique of impaction allografting may be applied to any situation where bone is deficient. However, in practice, it is most easily applied to a case where the proximal femur still comprises an intact tube, albeit a very weakened one. Should the surgeon wish to use the technique to reconstruct more dramatic deficiencies, some form of material will be required to seal off the deficient areas before impaction can be performed. The technique of impaction allografting has shown good early results[7], and is based on earlier work undertaken in Sweden, though applied to the acetabulum[8]. Good clinical, and radiological (Figure 8.1), results can be obtained.

## Before the operation

As with all revision procedures, careful preoperative planning is essential. It is vital the surgeon be aware if infection is present before operation begins as this may be an indication for a two-stage procedure. A thorough history and examination, combined with isotope scanning (gallium or indium), erythrocyte sedimentation rate (ESR), and C-reactive protein estimations (CRP) are thus advisable. Hip aspiration, under general or local anaesthetic, may also be undertaken if considered

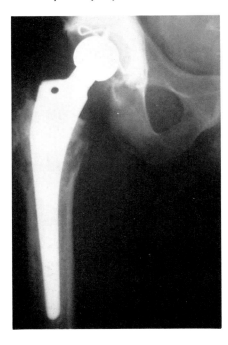

**Figure 8.1** Cemented, impaction allografting 2 years after surgery. The patient is fully weight-bearing. Note the good, vertical alignment of the femoral component in the presence of integrating allograft.

appropriate. Allograft tissue is essentially dead tissue, in itself an infection risk, and so every effort should be made to identify and eliminate infection before allografting is performed. Preoperative X-rays are also important. These should show not only the prosthesis, but well beyond its tip on both anteroposterior and lateral views. This permits the surgeon to anticipate likely difficulties at operation, and hence avoid them. For example, is the stem in varus? If so, it is likely that any blind use of cement drills can lead to intraoperative cortical perforation. A number of other questions are likely to face the revision surgeon. These may be as follows:

• What design of component is currently in place, and does our operating theatre have the wherewithal to remove it?

With so many designs on the market today, it is quite likely that the revision surgeon will be faced with having to remove a component he has never before used, and may never have seen. So-called 'universal' extractors do exist, but it is wise to ensure that the prosthesis manufacturers are also approached to ensure that all necessary equipment is available.

• Is it necessary to remove both components and what am I going to use in its place?

Again, this problem must be addressed beforehand. It may be necessary to prepare custom components to order, and it may be possible to revise only one side of the failed replacement. It is not always necessary to reconstruct both components in modern revision surgery. However, the operator should err on the side of caution and revise both sides if there is ever any doubt.

• Can I use the original components after bony reconstruction?

Horrifying though it may sound, there are occasions when it is permissible to reinsert the original components after bony reconstruction, though this particular situation is rare. For example, the patient may be very elderly and frail, only one side of the replacement may have failed, with failure being as a result of bone stock loss rather than prosthetic malfunction. For a quick, simple, safe procedure, replacement of the original components, after bony reconstruction, may be considered.

• Finally, is the patient sufficiently strong to tolerate an impaction allografting procedure?

Impaction allografting, successful though it may be, does require a lengthy period on crutches following surgery. If a patient is likely to be unable to tolerate up to three months limited weight-bearing, it is perhaps best to avoid impaction allografting as an option.

## The operation

The basic principle of impaction grafting is to achieve tightly packed bone against a clean endosteal surface. Sufficient quantity of allograft should thus be available and the surgeon, though being cautious, should not be timid.

No one approach is appropriate for an impaction procedure. However, the surgeon should ensure that exposure is sufficiently wide to allow safe removal of the failed component, a good view down the femoral shaft, with thorough cleaning and debridement of the canal. The endosteal surface needs to be cleaned to a point beyond the most distal lytic area visible on X-Ray. There is no absolute requirement to remove the distal cement plug. This sometimes acts as an effective cement restrictor for the revision operation. It also provides purchase for a guide wire, should this be used as part of the impaction grafting instrumentation.

Once the femoral canal is clear, the surgeon should then reconstruct any cortical deficiencies. Calcar reconstruction is best performed after trial reduction. Such deficiencies may be reconstructed with wire mesh, or with strut allografts, or a combination of the two. The aim is to achieve an intact tube into which morsellized allograft can be compressed. The quantity of allograft required is variable, but a minimum of three femoral heads can be expected. Many professional tissue banks now provide pre-morsellized bone, eliminating the requirement for bone milling in theatre. This is a valuable time-saving device, and also ensures sterility. Should a professional facility be used, a minimum of 120 g of morsellized allograft should be requested (1 femoral head equivalent = 40 g) for the 'average' femoral reconstruction. To have too little bone present can tempt the surgeon to incompletely impact. This, in turn, may lead to premature failure. Allograft chip size is hotly debated in revision circles. No one size is essential. However, the chips should be large enough to ensure they do not disappear down the sucker at surgery, whilst being sufficiently small to permit easy impaction. A chip size of 0.5 cm is reasonable in this respect. Frozen allograft bone appears to be the most versatile. Freeze-dried tissue can be used, but requires reconstitution and can be more difficult to handle.

Once the femoral canal has been cleaned, and distal plugging obtained, impaction may then begin. This is performed, from distal to proximal, in a slow and steady manner. It is a useful precaution to surround the impacted area of canal with cerclage wires, or bone holders, to minimize the chance of intraoperative fracture. Specialist impactor systems exist, but whether or not these are used, the principle remains the same. The femoral canal is gradually filled with sequentially impacted allograft morsels from distal to proximal, using a gradually increasing size of impactor. Should specialist impactors not be available, the technique can be performed using standard femoral rasps. The surgeon should reach a point where a trial stem can be inserted into the impacted bone, but cannot be removed manually. No motion should be visible when the trial is twisted within the canal. When the trial is removed, a new femoral canal can be seen, lined with compressed allograft bone.

Despite tight impaction, a standard scrub and squirt technique is obviously impractical prior to cementation. However, in order to obtain as dry a surface as possible a small swab may be passed gently down the new canal. A venting tube is then passed down inside the swab, preventing any direct contact between venting tube and impacted allograft. This is left in place whilst cement mixing is performed. Once the venting tube and swab are removed, a clean, dry, inner allograft surface will be seen. Tube and swab must be removed carefully, to ensure that the impacted allograft surface is not dragged upwards. Cement is then inserted, under pressure, in a routine manner, using a cement gun. Again, this is performed from distal to proximal. Tapered gun nozzles are available if required.

As has now become routine in many units, prosthetic insertion is delayed until the cement has reached a more doughy, manageable consistency. In the presence of impacted allograft this is vitally important as pressurization serves to impact the graft still further. One would imagine that femoral component insertion is simple; it is not. During the impaction process the orifice of the new canal is easy to see. After cementation it is lost from view, unless some form of guide wire system is used. It is therefore possible to disrupt the allograft mantle during component insertion unless great care and caution are taken. Once inserted, however, pressure is maintained on the component until cement curing is complete.

## After the operation

Postoperative management varies widely. For example, the initial recommendation for patients undergoing impacted acetabular allografting was for 6 weeks' strict bed rest after surgery. However, for most cases of femoral impaction the patient may be mobilized at 48 hours. Non-weight-bearing, or very limited partial weight-bearing, should be encouraged for a minimum of 12 weeks after operation. For more major reconstructions, a longer period of bed rest, and more prolonged non-weight-bearing, is advisable.

Throughout the surgical episode, antibiotic cover and anti-deep vein thrombosis (DVT) treatment is provided. It is also wise that a specimen of the allograft used be sent for bacteriological analysis during surgery, as a precaution should graft contamination have occurred. Graft contamination is a genuine problem, particularly for orthopaedic departmental bone banks[9].

# Results

Exeter, in the United Kingdom, has perhaps the greatest and longest global experience of femoral impaction allografting in revision surgery. There, more than 330 cases have been performed, some patients now being reviewed for up to 7½ years[10]. Results appear excellent, with a cohort of 56 hips followed for 18–49 months showing few complications and good evidence of incorporation of the graft[7]. Post-mortem retrieval has revealed direct contact between new living bone and cement[11], with a cement–tissue interface resembling that seen after primary cemented arthroplasty. Irrespective of the degree of bone stock loss, favourable reports are now beginning to appear from other centres, though intra-operative femoral fracture is a recognized risk[12]. Some are also recommending cementless revision in association with impaction allografting, though results are currently only short term[13]. There is some laboratory work to support this approach[14].

# References

1. Pellici, P.M., Wilson, P.D., Sledge, C.B. et al. (1985) Long-term results of revision total hip replacement: a follow-up report. *J. Bone Joint Surg.*, **67A**, 513–516.
2. Kershaw, C.J., Atkins, R.M., Dodd, C.A.F., and Bulstrode, C.J.K. (1991) Revision total hip arthroplasty for aseptic failure: a review of 276 cases. *J. Bone Joint Surg.*, **73B**, 564–568.
3. Retpen, J.B., Varmarken, J.-B., Rock, N.D. and Steen-Jensen, J. (1992) Unsatisfactory result after repeated revision of hip arthroplasty. *Acta Orthop. Scand.*, **63**, 120–127.
4. Schuller, H.M., Marti, R.K. and Besselaar, P.P. (1988) Aseptic failure in revision hip replacement. *Acta Orthop. Scand.*, Suppl. **227**, 34–35.
5. Rubash, H.E. and Harris, W.E. (1988) Revision of non-septic, loose, cemented femoral components using modern cementing techniques. *J. Arthroplasty*, **3**, 241–248.
6. Dohmae, Y., Bechtol, J.E., Sherman, R.E. et al. (1988) Reduction in cement-bone interface shear strength between primary and revision arthroplasty. *Clin. Orthop.*, **236**, 214–220.
7. Gie, G.A., Linder, L., Ling, R.S.M. et al. (1993) Impacted cancellous allografts and cement for revision hip arthroplasty. *J. Bone Joint Surg.*, **75B**, 14–21.
8. Slooff, T.J.J.H., Huiskes, R., van Horn, J. and Lemmens, A.J. (1984) Bone grafting in total hip replacement for acetabular protrusio. *Acta Orthop. Scand.*, **55**, 593–596.
9. Chapman, P. and Villar, R. (1992) The bacteriology of bone allografts. *J. Bone Joint Surg.*, **74B**, 398–399.
10. Gie, G.A. (1995) Revision hip replacement: impaction bone grafting. *Current Medical Literature*, **8(1)**, 3–5.
11. Ling, R.S.M., Timperley, A.J. and Linder, L. (1993) Histology of impaction cancellous grafting in the femur. *J. Bone Joint Surg.*, **73B**, 693–696.
12. Lucht, U. and Andersen, K. (1995) Impacted cancellous allografts and cement in revision hip arthroplasty. *J. Bone Joint Surg.*, **77B**, Suppl. 106–107.
13. Solgaard, S. and Retpen, J.B. (1995) Impaction allografting with cementless fixation. *J. Bone Joint Surg.*, **77B**, Suppl I; 98–99.
14. McDonald, D.J., Fitzgerald, R.H. Jr and Chao, E.Y.S (1988) The enhancement of fixation of a porous-coated femoral component by autograft and allograft in the dog. *J. Bone Joint Surg.*, **70A**, 728–737.

# 9

# Reconstruction of the femur

Allan E. Gross

Revision surgery for loose hip and knee implants is now a major part of any orthopaedic surgical programme, and its volume is going to increase. Loose cemented hip and knee prostheses, particularly in the multiply revised implant, are associated with loss of bone stock due to wear particles and the loose cement acting as an abrasive[1–9]. Wear particles may cause bone lysis even in the presence of stable cemented or uncemented components[10,11]. Also each time a revision is carried out, the surgery itself leads to some loss of bone stock. The symptomatic loose knee or hip prosthesis with associated loss of bone stock is going to continue to be a standard orthopaedic problem occupying a significant portion of the surgical resources of any orthopaedic division that performs implant surgery. The problem, therefore, must be dealt with if orthopaedic surgeons are going to continue replacing arthritic joints.

There are surgical alternatives for this problem. Excision arthroplasty may be acceptable but not when the bone loss is extensive[12,13]. Arthrodesis is difficult to achieve and results in excessive shortening if bone loss is extensive[14]. The use of tumour or custom implants where bone is replaced by metal may be acceptable in low demand patients but there are certain disadvantages. The large tumour implants may require the use of cement in the host bone, which can no longer provide the rough lattice necessary for good cement techniques. A stress riser is created at the junction of host bone and implant with both cemented and uncemented implants[15–21]. The prosthesis does not provide a biological anchorage for host bone and muscle.

Restoration of bone stock in association with a relatively conventional implant offers a more normal gradation of forces from the prosthesis to host bone. The reattachment of bone and muscle is possible. The implant may be of a more conventional design and may be less expensive. Restoration of bone stock also allows the surgeon to use uncemented or cemented implants, and most importantly, it may allow further revisions if necessary in the future.

Bone stock may be replenished by the patient's own bone or allograft bone. Using the patient's own bone is only applicable where a minimal amount of bone is required. Allograft bone offers quality and quantity and is applicable in certain situations where major defects exist, i.e. proximal femoral or major pelvic column loss. There are also the obvious advantages to leaving the patient's iliac crest intact.

There are, of course, certain disadvantages to using allograft bone. The problems of disease transmission are discussed elsewhere in this book. Banked bone is not always readily available but is becoming increasingly more so. Allograft bone has certain biological problems. It is not as osteoinductive as autograft bone and non-unions may result[22]. This can be alleviated by autografting host allograft junctions and obtaining rigid fixation. Resorption of allograft bone, particularly solid fragment grafts, may lead to failure[23,24]. This of course, may also occur with autograft bone but the process probably is slower. There may be problems like fracture or fragmentation of solid fragment grafts if the biomechanics of the reconstruction are not correct or if the patient is of too high a demand. This problem applies to both auto and allografts. Whatever the problems are, however, there is no question that we are facing a large population of patients who are going to need restoration of bone stock before further revision surgery can be performed.

## Classification of bone defects

It is important to have a functional and relatively simple classification of bone deficits associated with loose hip implants. There are more complicated classifications in the literature[25,26] but we have found that all of our grafts can be fitted into the following classification:

### Femoral side defects

1. Intraluminal — the canal is widened but the cortex is still intact and thought to be strong enough to support an implant.
2. Cortical —
   (a) Cortical non-circumferential — these are cortical defects that require only strut grafts
   (b) Circumferential — these are classified into:
      i. Calcar — < 3 cm in length
      ii. Proximal femur (large fragment) — > 3 cm in length

These bone defects can be classified, in most cases, by plain X-rays (routine views, Judet views)[27]; CAT scans may be helpful, particularly when first starting to do these types of reconstructions, but they are not usually necessary.

Infection is determined by routine blood work, gallium and technetium scans, preoperative hip aspiration, and Gram's stains at the time of surgery.

## Surgical techniques

In our hospital, all revision requiring the use of allograft bone are done in a laminar flow operating room with body exhaust systems. If there is preoperative evidence of infection or any suggestion at the time of surgery (even with a negative Gram's stain), the surgery is staged for any revision requiring the use of allograft bone.

Any allograft bone is brought into the operating room at the beginning of the case, unwrapped, cultured, and immersed in warm Betadine. The bone is obtained from our own bone bank, where it has been deep frozen at −70°C after being irradiated with 2.5 megarads.

## Surgical approach

The surgical approach is either transgluteal[28] or transtrochanteric. The transtrochanteric approach is used most commonly because of the need for extensive exposure and also because, in many cases, there is a pre-existing trochanteric non-union.

The large fragment proximal femoral grafts should be done via the transtrochanteric approach and the trochanteric fragment should be kept as long as possible so that it will unite and so it will also reinforce the allograft. The proximal femur is exposed by reflecting the vastus lateralis off the septum anteriorly, being careful not to strip any residual bone of its soft tissue completely.

A Steinmann pin is inserted into the iliac crest as a reference point to adjust leg lengths. The distance from the pin to the rough line (insertion of the vastus lateralis) is recorded prior to dislocation.

**Table 9.1  Femoral side defects**

| Cavitary defect | Intraluminal graft with long-stem press-fit femoral component or cemented femoral component |
|---|---|
| Structural defect | *Non-cylindrical*: cortical strut graft<br>*Cylindrical*: proximal femoral allograft with cemented femoral component; cement may be used in allograft but not in host |

## Femur (see Table 9.1, Figure 9.1)

The acetabulum is reconstructed first in order that the length of the femoral allograft can be determined.

We use long-stem femoral components and therefore we do not hesitate to cut a window for controlled cement removal and reaming. If a proximal femoral allograft is to be performed, then the residual proximal femur is split distally to good bone. As much soft tissue as possible is left attached to the residual bone for later use as a vascularized bone graft. The cement is then removed.

The distal host femur is then reamed gently over a guide wire to assess canal size for the implant rather than to enlarge the canal. When the reamers are at a size that definite reaming is taking place, then the diameter of implant is selected. The allograft, which is either proximal femur or tibia, is then reamed and broached until a good fit for the implant is achieved. It is important not to over-

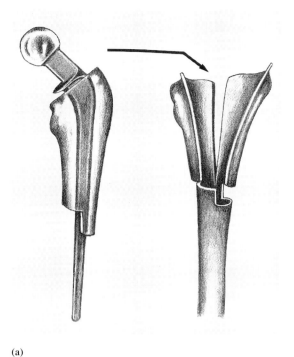

(a)

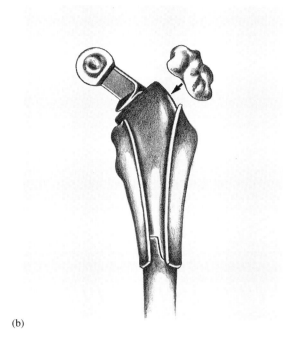

(b)

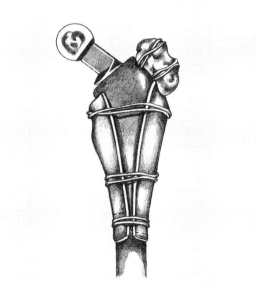

(c)

**Figure 9.1** Drawing of femoral reconstruction: a, The femoral allograft has been prepared and the step-cut made, and the femoral implant cemented into the allograft. The residual host femur has been split. b, The allograft and implant are seated in the bed of the host bone. c, The femoral implant is cemented into the allograft but not to the host. Fixation to the host is achieved by cerclage wires around the step-cut and wrapping residual host bone also with cerclage wires around the step-cut. The host bone helps with fixation and also provides a living bone autograft. Any autograft bone that is available should be applied to the junction of graft and host.

ream the allograft in order to get a press-fit of the femoral component into the host. The host canal is always larger than the allograft and therefore it may be impossible to get a press-fit into the host without over-reaming the allograft which would weaken it. We therefore cement the implant to the allograft and use a step-cut at the junction of host and allograft to gain stability rather than worry about the press-fit. The length of the allograft necessary is assessed *in vivo* by placing the femoral implant into the host bone and reducing it into the trial cup. The selected length depends on stability and leg length discrepancy. A Steinmann pin is inserted into the iliac crest and the distance from it to a fixed point on the femur is measured prior to dislocation of the hip. A step-cut of about 2 cm × 2 cm is carried out in the allograft (positive step) and in the host (negative step). Sometimes the host allograft junction is stable without a step-cut. Under these circumstances the step-cut is not necessary. If obtaining stability at the junction is difficult then cortical strut allografts can be cerclaged around the junction for additional fixation.

When the correct length of allograft is obtained

and the stability of the reconstruction is acceptable, the implant is cemented into the allograft after drill holes are made and wires are passed for trochanteric reattachment. It is very important to keep the cement off the interface that will oppose host bone. The allograft with the long stem femoral component cemented in place is inserted into the host and cerclage wire is used to stabilize the step-cut. The junction of host and allograft is also autografted by reamings or other host bone that is available. The residual host proximal femur is wrapped around the allograft and held by cerclaged

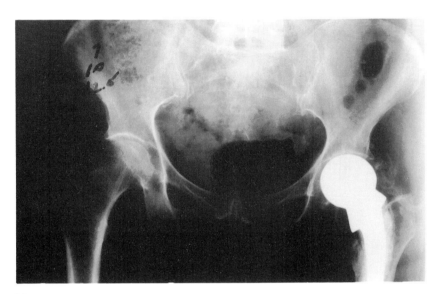

(a)

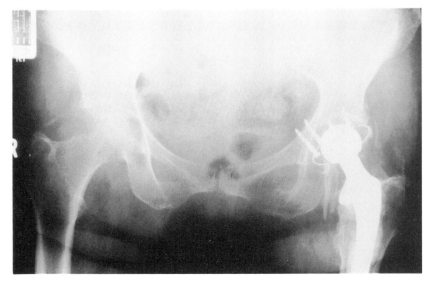

(b)

**Figure 9.2** Successful calcar a, Preoperative X-ray of left hip showing a cemented unipolar arthroplasty in a 65-year-old female. b, A.P. X-ray 7 years after a calcar allograft with implant cemented into allograft. The allograft is intact, has undergone some remodelling and the implant is stable.

wires. An attempt is made to bring these vascularized pieces distally to wrap around the osteotomy junction to encourage union.

We attempt to obtain a press-fit of the long stem femoral component but this is not crucial for success because once union is achieved at the osteotomy and the implant is cemented to the allograft, the femoral reconstruction is stabilized. It is our opinion that bone ingrowth is impossible to obtain in these multiply revised femoral reconstructions and, therefore, porous coating on the femoral component is not necessary. The implant is always cemented to the allograft.

Cortical strut allografts are used to reinforce windows or stress risers or may be used to stabilize osteotomy or allograft host junctions. They are wired into place and if possible their ends autografted to encourage union to host.

## Postoperative care

Prophylactic intravenous antibiotics are used for 5 days followed by 5 more days of oral antibiotics. We prefer a cephalosporin. If the patient is catheterized intraoperatively, we use gentamicin during the surgery and for the first 24 hours but then switch to septrin until the catheter is removed. Because of the extent of the surgery, we usually keep the patients on bed rest in abduction for 5 days. The patients are not allowed any weight bearing until union is obtained between allograft and host, usually at 3–6 months.

## Principles of surgery for femoral grafting

1. Use a wide exposure. Trochanteric osteotomy and reflection of the vastus lateralis off the anterior part of the femur offers the best and safest exposure. Do not hesitate to use windows which allow cement removal and safe controlled reaming. If a circumferential graft is to be used the residual host femur should be split and used as a vascularized wrap around graft to encourage allograft host union and to strengthen the allograft. Do not sacrifice or devascularize host bone for this reason.
2. The implant should be cemented into the allograft but not into the host. Cement strengthens the graft and theoretically delays vascularization and membrane formation. Grafts should be longer than 3 cm.

3. Rigid fixation must be achieved between allograft and host.
4. Autograft allograft host junction.
5. Do not use structural circumferential grafts unless necessary but if necessary use strong young bone.
6. Do not drill holes into the allograft except for trochanteric attachment.

## Results

In an earlier follow-up study of 32 calcar grafts (less than 3 cm in length) with an average follow-up of 4.36 years, 16 had uncemented implants and 16 cemented implants. We found that although these grafts seem to do well clinically, there was an unacceptable rate of implant subsidence (43%), and a resorption of over 50% in 40% of grafts that had uncemented implants. These calcar grafts did much better if they were cemented, lessening the incidence of resorption to 10%. We, however, now feel that there is no real indication for a graft less than 3 cm in length because that amount of length can be compensated for by the implant. When, however, short grafts are necessary, they should be cemented following the same principles as the long grafts (Figures 9.2, 9.3).

In an earlier study of our large proximal femoral grafts 40 grafts with an average follow-up of 36.6 months (range 29–83) were assessed clinically and radiologically[29]. A modified Harris scoring system was used with failure of the procedure being defined as (Table 9.2):

1. Failure to improve the hip score by at least 20 points,
2. The need for any further surgery related to the allograft.

The 40 hips in which large fragment grafts were used had an average preoperative score of 30.5 (range 6–58) and an average postoperative score of 65.8 (range 21–100), an average improvement of 35.3.

The average length of these grafts was 10.4 cm (range 3.5–17).

Radiographic evaluation was possible in only 37 of the 40 hips, because 3 failed shortly after operation. There was evidence of union between the allograft and the host bone in 30 of these 37 hips (81%). Bone bridging across a persistent defect was seen in 3 (8%). Stable non-union occurred in 1 (3%) and unstable non-union in 3 (8%).

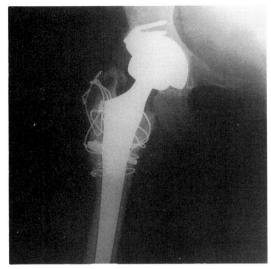

(a)

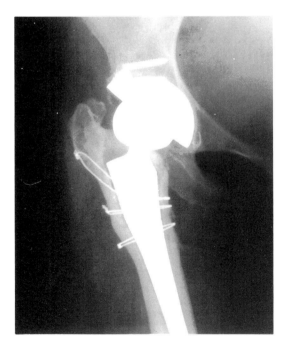

(b)

**Figure 9.3** Unsuccessful calcar allograft a, A.P. X-ray right hip showing a calcar allograft supporting an uncemented femoral implant in a 30-year-old female. b, A.P. X-ray at 2 years showing significant subsidence of the implant into allograft.

**Table 9.2    Hip rating**

| | |
|---|---|
| Pain | Deformity |
| 44 = None | Fixed Adduction |
| 40 = Slight | 1 = < 10 |
| 30 = Moderate, occasional | 0 = > 10 |
| 20 = Moderate | |
| 10 = Marked | Fixed Internal Rotation |
| 0 = Disabled | 1 = < 10 |
| | 0 = > 10 |
| Function | |
| Limp | Flexion Contracture |
| 11 = None | 1 = < 15 |
| 8 = Slight | 0 = > 15 |
| 5 = Moderate | |
| 0 = Severe | Leg Length Discrepancy |
| | 1 = < 3 cm |
| Support | 0 = > 3 cm |
| 11 = None | |
| 7 = Cane, long walks | Range of Motion |
| 3 = 1 Crutch | Flexion |
| 2 = 2 Canes | 1 = > 90 |
| 0 = 2 Crutches | 0 = < 90 |
| | |
| Distance Walked | Abduction |
| 11 = Unlimited | 1 = > 15 |
| 8 = 6 Blocks | 0 = < 15 |
| 5 = 3 Blocks | |
| 2 = Indoors | Adduction |
| 0 = Bed and chair | 1 = > 15 |
| | 0 = < 15 |
| Activities | |
| Stairs | External Rotation |
| 4 = Normally | 1 = > 30 |
| 2 = Without railing | 0 = < 30 |
| 1 = Any manner | |
| 0 = Unable | Internal Rotation |
| | 1 = > 15 |
| Shoes and Socks | 0 = < 15 |
| 4 = With ease | |
| 2 = With difficulty | Trendelenburg |
| 0 = Unable | 1 = Negative |
| | 0 = Positive |
| Sitting | |
| 4 = Any chair, 1 hours | |
| 2 = High chair | |
| 0 = Unable to sit comfortably | |
| | |
| Public Transportation | |
| 1 = Able to use | |
| 0 = Unable to use | |

One graft, 4 cm long, fragmented, but resorption of these large grafts was not seen. In 4 hips (11%) there was subsidence ranging from 0.5 to 1.5 cm (average 1). Gross failure of the construct did not occur.

In the 24 hips which had trochanteric osteotomies, bony radiological union occurred in 9 (38%) and stable fibrous union in 10 (42%). In 5 hips the trochanter displaced more than 1 cm.

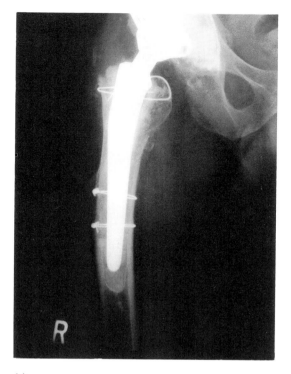

(a)

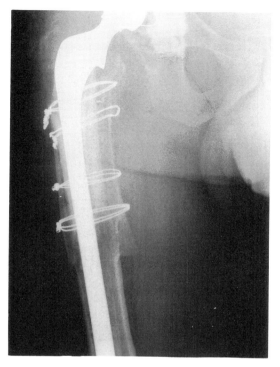

(b)

**Figure 9.4** Proximal femoral allograft. a, A.P. X-ray of right hip showing a loose femoral component with loss of proximal femoral bone stock in a 40-year-old male. b, A.P. X-ray right hip 7 years after proximal femoral allograft with femoral component cemented into allograft but not into host. The implant is stable and union between allograft and host is solid. The host bone is reinforcing but not replacing the allograft, and also helped in union between allograft and host.

In 4 hips the score failed to increase postoperatively by 20 points. These included 1 patient with chronic pain and venous insufficiency who subsequently underwent hip disarticulation and 1 case of symptomatic nonunion.

Four patients underwent resection arthroplasty, 3 for deep infection and 1 for recurrent dislocation. The latter patient had spina bifida and paralytic hip dysplasia.

There was 1 death, due to laceration of the external iliac vein during acetabular reconstruction.

The overall success rate was 80%. However, if 2 patients with high postoperative hip scores who also had high preoperative score were regarded as successful the rate improves to 85% (Figures 9.4, 9.5, 9.6).

Seven cortical strut grafts were also evaluated as part of that study[28]. They all united and remodelled. There was no subsidence of any prosthesis and no graft structural failure. One patient failed to increase his score by 20 points, giving a success rate of 86%.

As of July 1, 1993, 235 proximal femoral allografts have been used for revision arthroplasty of the hip with an average follow-up of 4.36 years and a range of 1–10 years; 176 grafts were cylindrical, 51 cortical struts and 8 intraluminal. Of the cylindrical grafts 32 were calcar grafts (less than 3 cm in length) and 144 were longer than 3 cm in length.

At the present time, all of our femoral grafts are longer than 3 cm and are simply called large fragment proximal femoral allograft. Of the 235 proximal femoral grafts including the calcar grafts with an average follow-up of 4.36 years there have been 17 revisions for a revision rate of 7%. Four femoral allografts required plating and bone grafting for non-union (all larger grafts). One calcar graft was revised because of resorption and 2 calcar grafts required revision for loose implants. Two femoral allografts were revised for infection, 7 for dislocation, and 1 for pain (all large proximal femoral grafts). All revisions were successful.

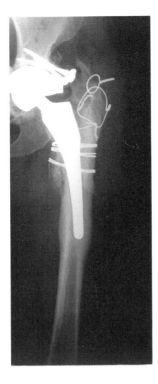

(a)

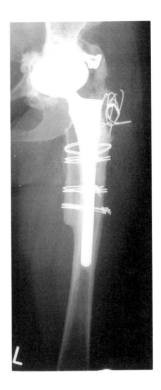

(b)

**Figure 9.5**  Cortical strut allograft. a, A.P. X-ray of left hip in 35-year-old female with loose uncemented femoral implant and fracture of medial femoral cortex. The cup is also loose.

b, A.P. X-ray 3 years after medial cortical strut allograft. A combination of the cortical strut allograft and host bone support the implant.

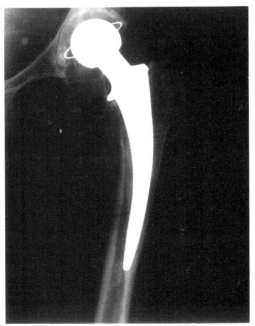

(a)

**Figure 9.6**  Cortical strut allograft. a, A.P. X-ray left hip in a 55-year-old female with a loose cemented femoral component and erosion of lateral femoral cortex.

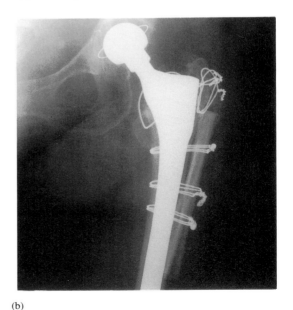

(b)

b, A.P. X-ray 3 months after reconstruction with a cortical strut allograft and long stem uncemented component.

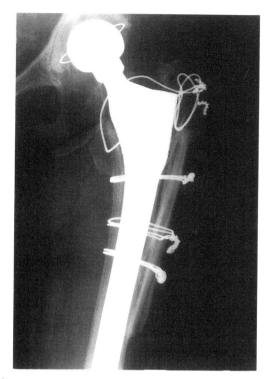

(c)

c, A.P. X-ray 2 years later showing union and remodelling of the cortical strut.

# References

1. Freeman, M.A.R., Bradley, G.W. and Revell, P.A. (1982) Observations upon the interface between bone and poly-methylmethacrylate cement. *J. Bone Joint Surg.*, **64B**, 489.
2. Goldring, S.R., Schiller, A.I., Roelke, M.S. et al. (1986) Formation of a synovial-like membrane at the bone cement interface. *Arthritis Rheum.*, **29**, 836.
3. Goldring, S.R., Schiller, A.L., Roelke, M. et al. (1983) The synovial-like membrane at the bone cement interface in loose total hip replacements and its proposed role in bone lysis. *J. Bone Joint Surg.*, **65A**, 575.
4. Goodman, S.B., Schatzker, J., Sumner-Smith, G. et al. (1985) The effect of polymethylmethacrylate on bone; an experimental study. *Arch. Orthop. Trauma Surg.*, **104**, 150.
5. Howie, D., Oakeshott, R., Manthy, B. et al. (1987) Bone resorption in the presence of polyethylene wear particles. *J. Bone Joint Surg.*, **69B**, 165.
6. Jasty, M.J., Floyd, W.E., Schiller, A.L. et al. (1986) Localized osteolysis in stable, non-septic total hip replacement. *J. Bone Joint Surg.*, **68A**, 912.
7. Linder, L., Lindberg, L. and Carlsson, A. (1983) Aseptic loosening of hip prostheses. *Clin. Orthop.*, **175**, 93.
8. Pazzaglia, U.E., Ceciliani, L., Wilkinson, M.J. et al. (1985) Involvement of metal particles in loosening of metal-plastic total hip prostheses. *Arch. Orthop. Trauma Surg.*, **104**, 164.
9. Revell, P.A., Weightman, B., Freeman, M.A.R. et al. (1978) The production and biology of polyethylene wear debris. *Arch. Orthop. Trauma Surg.*, **91**, 167.
10. Schmalzried, P., Jasty, M. and Harris, W.H. (1992) Periprosthetic bone loss in total hip arthroplasty. *J. Bone Joint Surg.*, **74A**, 849–863.
11. Maloney, W.J., Jasty, M., Harris, W.H. et al. (1990) Endosteal erosion in association with stable uncemented femoral components. *J. Bone Joint Surg.*, **72A**, 1025–1034.
12. Harris, W.H. and White, R.E. Jr (1982) Resection arthroplasty for non-septic failure of total hip arthroplasty. *Clin. Orthop.*, **171**, 62.
13. Grauer, J.D., Amstutz, H.C., O'Carroll, F. et al. (1989) Resection arthroplasty of the hip. *J. Bone Joint Surg.*, **71A**, 669–678.
14. Kostuik, J. and Alexander, D. (1984) Arthrodesis for failed arthroplasty of the hip. *Clin. Orthop.*, **188**, 173–182.
15. Chao, E.Y.S. and Sim, F.H. (1992) Composite fixation of salvage prostheses for the hip and the knee. *Clin. Orthop.*, **276**, 91.
16. Unwin, P.S., Cobb, J.P. and Walker, P.S. (1993) Distal femoral arthroplasty using custom-made prostheses; the first 218 cases. *J. Arthroplasty*, **8:3**, 259–268.
17. Blunn, G.W., Hua, J., Wait, M.E. and Walker, P.S. (1991) Correlation of stress distribution with bony remodelling in retrieved femora with proximal femoral replacement. In *Complications of Limb Salvage* (K. Brown, ed.) ISOLS, Montreal, pp. 445–450.
18. Markel, M.D., Gottsauner-Wolf, F., Rock, M.G. et al. (1991) A mechanical comparison of six methods of proximal femoral replacement. In *Complications of Limb Salvage* (K. Brown, ed.) ISOLS, Montreal, pp. 75–80.
19. Zehr, R.J., Heare, T., Enneking, W.F. et al. (1991) Allograft prosthesis composite vs. megaprosthesis in proximal femoral reconstruction. In *Complications of Limb Salvage* (K. Brown, ed.) ISOLS, Montreal, pp. 91–103.
20. Unwin, P.S., Cobb, J.P., Walker, P.S. et al. (1991) Loosening in cemented femoral prostheses: a study of 668 tumour cases. In *Complications of Limb Salvage* (K. Brown, ed.) ISOLS, Montreal, pp. 133–137.
21. Wipperman, B., Zwipp, H., Sturm, J. et al. (1991) Complications of endoprosthetic proximal femoral replacement. In *Complications of Limb Salvage* (K. Brown, ed.) ISOLS, Montreal, pp. 143–146.
22. Czitrom, A., Gross, A., Langer, F. et al. (1988) Bone banks and allografts in community practice. *Instructional Course Lectures American Academy of Orthopaedic Surgeons*, **37**, 24–31.
23. Oakeshott, R.D., Morgan, D.A.F., Zukor, D.J. et al. (1987) Revision total hip arthroplasty with osseous allograft reconstruction. *Clin. Orthop.*, **225**, 37–61.
24. Oakeshott, R.D., McAuley, J.P., Gross, A.E. et al. (1989) Allograft reconstruction in revision total hip surgery. In *Bone Transplantation* (M. Aebi and P. Regazzoni, eds) Berlin: Springer-Verlag; pp. 265–273.
25. Gustilo, R.D., and Pasternak, H.S. (1988) Revision total hip arthroplasty with a titanium ingrowth prosthesis and bone grafting for failed cemented femoral component loosening. *Clin. Orthop.*, **235**, 111–119.
26. D'Antonio, J.A., Capello, W.N. and Borden, L.S. (1989) Classification and management of acetabular abnormalities in total hip arthroplasty. *Clin. Orthop.*, **243**, 126–137.

27. Judet, R., Judet, J. and Letournel, E. (1964) Fractures of the acetabulum: classification and surgical approaches for open reduction. *J. Bone Joint Surg.*, **46A**, 1615–1646.

28. Hardinge, K. (1982) The direct lateral approach to the hip. *J. Bone Joint Surg.*, **64B**, 17–19.

29. Allan, D.G., Lavoie, G.J., McDonald S. et al. (1991) Proximal femoral allografts in revision hip arthroplasty. *J. Bone Joint Surg.*, **73B**, 235–238.

# 10

# Cemented femoral revision

Kevin Hardinge

Total hip arthroplasty is the most successful major elective procedure in the whole of surgery so that the need for revision is a source of disappointment for the patient and the surgeon. The onset of pain in a previously satisfactorily functioning arthroplasty can be due to loosening which is either aseptic or septic.

## Aseptic loosening

Aseptic loosening occurs as a remote complication where there has been a varying period of success-ful function, and is present without systemic symptoms. It presents as pain after function, tending to diminish with rest. There are no local signs of inflammation around the joint and there are no blood changes such as raised ESR or white cell count.

The radiographs may show demarcation of the cup which may be complete in the De Lee and Charnley zones I + II + III. (Figure 10.1). In this situation the cup is probably loose and if migration of the cup occurs, the cup is definitely loose (Figure 10.1)[1]. Demarcation of the stem has been categorized by Gruen[10]. If the demarcation is progressive, the

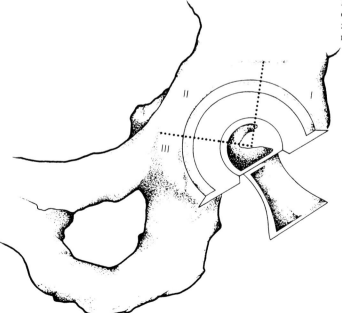

**Figure 10.1** De Lee and Charnley zones for demarcation of the cup. If demarcation is present in zones I, II, III the cup is probably loose. If migration of the cup occurs, loosening is confirmed.

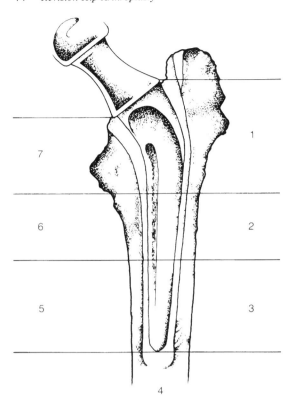

**Figure 10.2**   Thomas Gruen's (1979) zones for demarcation of the stem. If demarcation is present in all zones, loosening is probable. If subsidence occurs loosening is confirmed.

loosening is confirmed. Subsidence of the stem, incipient or actual, is usually preceded by fracture of the cement pedestal in the Gruen zone 4 (Figure 10.2).

## Septic loosening

All of the above clinical and radiological features may be present in septic loosening but the progression of the clinical course is much more rapid.

The inspection of the joint may show the classical signs of inflammation — rubor, turgor and dolor, and there may be signs of a systemic upset — pyrexia and malaise. The worst case scenario is a septicaemia with a positive blood culture, and the whole spectrum of bacteria–host response is dependent upon the virility of the organism and the ability of the patient to rally their immunological defences.

**Table 10.1   Conditions in which deep infection is seen more commonly**

| |
|---|
| Elderly |
| Anaemic |
| Malnutrition |
| Diabetes |
| Steroid medication |
| Re-operations — previous pin and plate |
| Prolonged surgery |
| Focal sepsis elsewhere |

**Table 10.2   Occurrence of immunological deficiency**

| |
|---|
| Extremes of age |
| Malnutrition |
| Malignancy |
| Immunosuppression |
| Metabolic disease (e.g. diabetes) |
| Collagen disease (rheumatoid arthritis) |
| Corticosteroids (ingestion of) |

Postoperative superficial and deep infections are known to occur more frequently when the host defences are impaired or immunological deficiency exists (Tables 10.1, 10.2).

## Diagnosis

When pain develops in a previously pain-free and stable total hip replacement, infection and mechanical loosening must be suspected.

Factors favouring an infection as the cause of pain are generalized systemic upset (high ESR, elevated WBC count), persistence of pain at rest, local signs of inflammation, history of intercurrent infection, and an association with steroids and rheumatoid arthritis. At an early stage there may or may not be demarcation of the implants. If demarcation of the implants is shown when the patient presents, it tends to indicate a low-grade infection (*Staphylococcus epidermidis*), particularly if the systemic disturbance is slight. On the other hand, severe systemic disturbance without signs of demarcation indicates a high-grade virulent infection (*Staphylococcus aureus*).

Joint aspiration can be useful in high-grade infections to identify the organism and its antibiotic sensitivity, but in low-grade infection there is a high incidence of false negatives.

The plain radiographs of the hip region will indicate, by the presence or absence of demarcation the extent of the infection. A septum of bone may have developed below the tip of the implant (when a femoral canal restrictor has been used), thus

**Table 10.3   Direct exchange revision**

| Requirements | Advantages | Disadvantages |
|---|---|---|
| General condition stable | Restoration of leg length | Bacteriology may be undetermined |
| Thorough debridement | Reduced hospitalisation | Fixation suboptimal |
| Bone must be sound | | Recurrence may occur |

**Table 10.4   Interval revision**

| Requirements | Advantages | Disadvantages |
|---|---|---|
| Removal of all components | Knowledge of bacteria present | Hospitalisation prolonged |
| Thorough debridement | Systemic disease settled | Limited goals procedure, leg discrepancy may persist<br>There may be a limp |

localizing the infected area, but the full extent may go beyond the upper third of the femur. A technetium bone scan will indicate the area of the skeleton in which there is increased blood flow[6, 7] — the infective process may extend to the lower end of the femur[8] and will determine the extent of the exploration necessary.

## Operative treatment

The goal, when revising a loosened cemented arthroplasty, is to restore the optimal fixation of the implant to ensure a full return of pain-free movement. The advantages, disadvantages of direct exchange revision as compared to interval revision is shown in Tables 10.3 and 10.4.

### Direct exchange revision

*Preparation of the skin*

It is the goal to eradicate all organisms and thus remove all potential pathogens (Table 10.5). The skin is a living tissue and in health contains organisms (Table 10.6), and these are considered to be normal skin commensals. In addition, other organisms are cultured from the skin that appear to be transiently present in health (Table 10.7). If the host's defences are impaired as in Table 10.2, it is conceivable that infection may take root that would otherwise not occur.

*Staphylococcus epidermidis* (*albus*) is present on the skin as a commensal but also causes deep infection in total joint replacements after a long incu-

bation period with no systemic disturbance. *S. epidermidis* is a heterogeneous group of staphylococci and micrococci that are all coagulase-negative and catalase-positive (Table 10.8).

The most common organism implicated in deep infection is *S. aureus*, which is found on the skin in 28% of healthy subjects.

**Table 10.5   Eradication of potential pathogens**

| Means | Result |
|---|---|
| Sterilization | Destroys all organisms and endospores |
| Disinfection | Destroys all organisms on inanimate objects |
| Antisepsis | Inhibits or destroys micro-organisms on living tissue |

**Table 10.6   Resident skin flora in health**

| Staphylococci | Micrococci | Diphtheroids |
|---|---|---|
| *Staphylococcus aureus* | | |
| | Gram-negative bacilli | |

**Table 10.7   Transient skin flora in health**

| | |
|---|---|
| *S. aureus* | Pseudomonas and other gram-negative organisms<br>Clostridial spores |

**Table 10.8   Staphylococcus epidermidis**

| Organism | Site |
|---|---|
| *S. hominis* | Skin |
| *S. epidermidis* | |
| *S. haemolyticus* | |
| *S. epidermidis* | Wound |
| *S. warneri* | |

The organism found in the wound at revision surgery by Charnley showed a predominance of *S. aureus* (Table 10.9). The low incidence of anaerobic infection or high rate of sterile cultures may represent inadequate bacteriological methodology since higher incidences have been found by other workers.

Our recent survey of 100 cases of revision shows a greater incidence of anaerobics (Table 10.10). Technique of surgery at the time of the initial operation and also the revision procedure will have an effect on the recurrence of infection.

The operating room environment is very important in determining the rate of postoperative infection in both primary and revision procedures (Table 10.11).

It is advisable to have an ultra-clean room for high-risk surgery. The number of colony-forming units per cubic metre in the operating room depends upon the type of ventilation employed (Table 10.11).

The importance of clean air was emphasized by Charnley who found a progressive reduction of deep sepsis with increasing the airflow over the operation site and thus diluting the bacteria (Table 10.11 and Figure 10.3)

Antibiotics were not used in this series, and a further reduction in the rate of infection was found in the Medical Research Council of Great Britain's trial as reported by Lidwell[2]. In this study, the combined effect of antibiotics, ultra-clean air, and body exhaust reduced the incidence of infection from 3.4% to 0.19% (Figure 10.3). These measures are equally important in the revision of deep sepsis where patients have already shown themselves to be susceptible to infection (Tables 10.12 and 10.13).

**Table 10.9   Infection in total hip replacement as found by Charnley**

| Organism | Percentage found |
|---|---|
| S. epidermidis | 4 |
| S. aureus | 33 |
| Anaerobic gram-positive cocci | 3 |
| Gram-negative bacilli | 12 |
| Anaerobic organisms | 0 |

**Table 10.10   Incidence of infecting organisms in 100 cases at Wrightington Hospital**

| Organism | Incidence (%) |
|---|---|
| S. epidermidis | 35 |
| S. aureus | 16 |
| Aerobic gram-positive cocci | 21 |
| Gram-negative bacilli | 7 |
| Anaerobic organisms | 15 |

**Table 10.11   Colony-forming units (CFU) per cubic metre**

| Type of ventilation | No CFU per c m |
|---|---|
| Conventional operating room | 180 |
| Horizontal box without body exhaust | 51 |
| Vertical flow with wall and body exhaust | 0.4 |

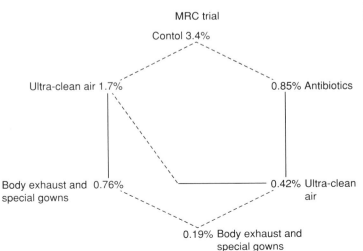

**Figure 10.3**   Reduction of infection, the various improvements observed by Lidwell in the M.R.C. Trial[2].

**Table 10.12   Contributing and preventative factors in wound infection**

| Contributing factors | Preventative factors |
| --- | --- |
| Previous surgery | |
| Previous infection in operative area | Diagnose coexisting local infection, ESR aspiration, biopsy |
| Coexisting local infection | |
| Decreased local vascularity (scarring) | |
| Skin lacerations, abrasions, blisters | |
| Skin bacteria (i.e. *S. epidermidis*) | Avoid surgery in presence of skin disease |
| Skin disease (e.g. psoriasis, steroids, atrophy) | Avoid shaving to prevent abrasions<br>Careful skin antisepsis<br>Repeated washings with proven antimicrobial (chlorhexidine, povidone-iodine), defatting solvent ether, acetone |
| Length of surgery (e.g. 2 h) | Minimize operating time |
| Implants | |
| Wound drying | |
| Haematoma and seroma | Observe careful surgical technique<br>Careful retraction, dissection and haemostasis |
| Defective wound healing | Minimize dead space<br>Irrigate frequently<br>Debride necrotic tissue<br>Meticulous wound closure<br>Suction drainage |

**Table 10.13   Factors increasing and reducing infection in the operating room environment**

| Factors increasing infection | Factors reducing infection |
| --- | --- |
| Contact bacterial contamination | Eliminate contact contamination |
| Break in sterile technique | Observe correct room cleansing procedure |
| Perforation in glove, gown or drape | Recognize and avoid breaks in sterile procedures |
| Soaked gown or drape | |
| Contaminated instruments or implants | |
| Inadequate air conditioning | Improve air conditioning |
| Dirty or inefficient filter | Check filter efficiency |
| Low air exchange rates | Check air flow patterns<br>Air exchange minimum 30–60 per hour |
| High temperature | Optimal temperature 70°F |
| High or low humidity | Optimal humidity, 50% |
| Negative operating room pressure | Positive pressure gradient from operating room to corridor |

In many cases it is not possible to decide if the loosening is aseptic or is due to an organism of low virulence. Attempted joint aspiration may fail to give a positive culture but swabs taken at operation are positive.

There will now be described a technique which is used in ambiguous cases, so that the organisms, if present, can be eradicated. This technique combines a respect for high-grade bacteriology with attention to low-grade hygiene, which can also be important.

*Hygienic considerations*

The hip is exposed using a trochanteric osteotomy with the patient in the supine position as this allows a wide exposure of the hip region. The hip is dislocated and swabs are taken of the joint fluid. It is a goal of direct exchange revision (der) to eradicate all organisms from the operation site and to create the ideal situation for successful implantation of the new prosthesis. The bone will vary in

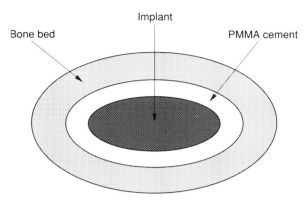

**Figure 10.4**   Schematic diagram showing the tissue planes to be considered in revision of total joint replacement.

its consistency. It may be friable as a result of chronic infection and quite unsuitable for der. In these cases it is often better to temporize with an interval Girdlestone operation until the bone tex-

ture improves (Figure 10.17, 10.18d and 10.18e). A schematic diagram (Figure 10.4) shows the tissue and implant planes in a perfectly stable implant.

In loosening of implants, the added factor is the development of a layer of connective tissue between the implant (stem and cement mantle) and the bone bed. If the loosening is sterile the connective tissue layer is quite dry and fibrous. If, however, there is an element of infection present, the soft-tissue granulation layer may be profuse, friable, wet and inflamed (Figure 10.5). All of these granulation tissues must be removed and it is a basic hygienic consideration to sterilize all stages of the debridement with copious amounts of topical antimicrobial (Figure 10.6). Chlorhexidine contains small amounts of cetrimide that acts as a detergent which facilitates removal of the 'film' that can encapsulate organisms.

The organisms are now exposed to the activity of povidone-iodine.

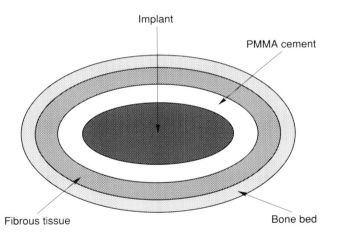

**Figure 10.5**   Schematic diagram of an infected total joint replacement. A thick layer of fibrous tissue has developed between the bone bed and the implant. This may show obvious signs of inflammation being friable and moist.

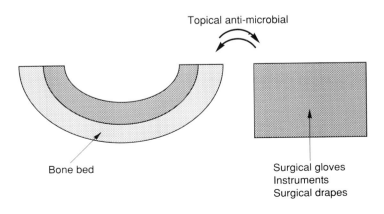

**Figure 10.6**   Removal of fibrous tissues must include copious lavage with topical antimicrobial to ensure that the circuit of organism from the operative site to the instrument tray is broken.

*Povidone-iodine*

The povidone-polymer effectively traps iodine and releases it in small amounts at a defined rate. The oxidizing agent used in the standard Betadine antiseptic solution is potassium iodate and the degree of oxidation can be kept constant by maintaining the pH constant at 5.8, i.e. the rate of oxidation is pH dependent.

The addition of iodate produces iodine (I) by 'mopping-up' the iodine ions ($I^+$) produced in the ageing process.

The $H^+$ ions generated means that the solution becomes more acidic with age. Reduced microbicidal efficiency and increased incidence of pH related side effects with age have hitherto been a potential problem in commercially available aqueous iodine solution.

It reacts with hydrocarbon in solution forming RI and $I_2$ and releasing $I^+$ ions. RI is microbicidally inactive. $I^-$ is inactive and this in itself goes on to consume more $I_2$ causing the production of $I_3$, which is also inactive.

## Preparation of the acetabulum

The cup is removed using an osteome that is curved on the flat[9]. It is usually possible to pass a curved osteome, that is straight in section, around the cup to remove it with its surrounding cement mantle.

The acetabulum is curetted of all its granulations and raw bleeding bone obtained that will take a good cement impregnation. A large swab impregnated with aqueous Betadine is placed in the acetabulum to sterilize it, preparatory to introducing the cement. These are the cases with an intact acetabular rim and intact floor (Figure 10.7).

There may be defects of the floor of the acetabulum or its rim (which have been classified by D'Antonio et al.[12]. Floor defects where there is an intact rim can be dealt with by a simple mesh technique (Figure 10.8 a, b).

The mesh is cut in radial sections so that it can be impressed into a hemisphere. A trial insertion will ensure that the edges of the mesh can be overlapped onto the acetabular rim (Figure 10.9 a, b, c and 10.10)

A suitable mix of cement, usually 2 packs, is inserted into the mesh and the cup is pressed onto the complex so that the flange engages with the mesh acetabular ring overlap, (Figure 10.11)

A flanged socket is pushed onto the mesh to ensure that the flange engages with the mesh 'mesh acetabular ring overlap'. (Figure 10.12).

Continuous pressure is kept on the complex whilst the cement is polymerizing to ensure that a one-piece acetabulum is produced. Because the cement possesses elasticity, it is usually permissible to permit partial weight-bearing early in the postoperative period.

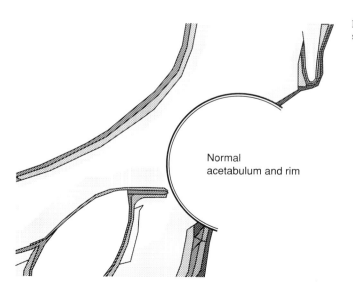

**Figure 10.7** Topographic diagram of hemipelvis showing acetabulum with intact floor and intact rim.

Normal
acetabulum and rim

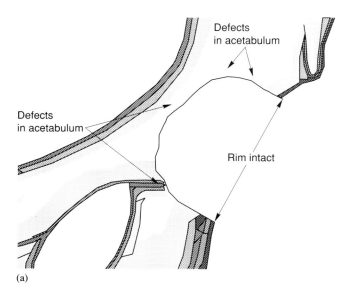

Defects
in acetabulum

Defects
in acetabulum

Rim intact

(a)

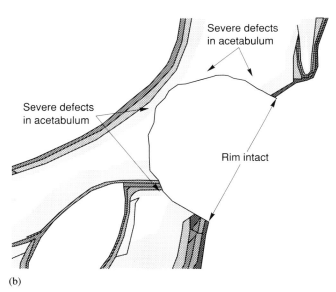

Severe defects
in acetabulum

Severe defects
in acetabulum

Rim intact

(b)

**Figure 10.8**  a, Topographic diagram of hemipelvis showing defects of the floor, the rim is still intact. b, Topographic diagram of hemipelvis showing severe defects of floor, but rim is still intact.

## Preparation of the femur

Cement drills are used to reduce the cicatrix of cement. If infection is present the cement–bone interface may be friable.

The cement mantle is usually irregular with the diamond-shaped stems or Charnley rectangular stem, and drilling and gouge cement thinning will produce a clearance. If the cement is firmly fixed to the bone it is not necessary to completely remove it but it should be sterilised as far as possible with topical antimicrobials (aqueous Betadine).

The object is to produce a conical mantle that will allow insertion of the revision stem. A useful conformity exists between the cavity produced by the drills and the Frustoconical stem. Drills of gradually increasing size are used to reduce the cement mantle (Figure 10.13a, b, c). At all stages of the revision, the operating site is washed with copious amounts of topical anti-microbial (aqueous Betadine).

It is important to avoid torsion on the femur with the larger drills to prevent fracture of the femur. It is preferable to use hand-powered tools and thus

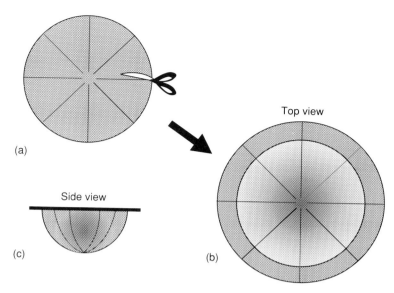

**Figure 10.9** Mesh used to reinforce severe defects of the floor of the acetabulum. The mesh is cut in a radial fashion as in (b) with the sections not reaching the centre. The sectors are overlapped when they are formed over a dome to fashion a hemisphere (c).

Top view

Side view

(a)

(c)

(b)

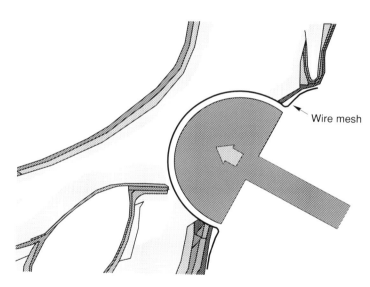

Wire mesh

**Figure 10.10** The mesh hemisphere is introduced to the defective floor at the acetabulum, and the peripheral flaps are allowed to overlap the intact acetabular rim. Fit is ensured by the dome pusher.

avoid excessive torsion by 'feeling' the resistance of the bone. In passing the drills down the femur, jamming may occur. If hand-held braces are being used, it is possible to feel that the turning of the drill is becoming more laboured before jamming occurs. It is imperative to avoid excessive torsion because the weakened bone may fracture. If the surgeon is using, for example, a 14 mm drill and it jams it is important to follow the following sequence:

1. remove the drill
2. wash out the cavity

3. go back to a smaller drill
4. ensure that the cavity is cleared by passage of the smaller drill
5. wash out the cavity
6. start again with the larger drill
7. ensure that you have gentle full rotations at the upper end of the femoral cavity
8. proceed slowly and gently down the cavity, ensuring always that you have a full rotation.

It is essential that the drills are kept sharp, as they can become blunted with many usages.

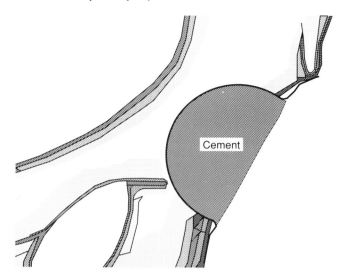

**Figure 10.11**  A bolus of cement is introduced into the mesh hemisphere.

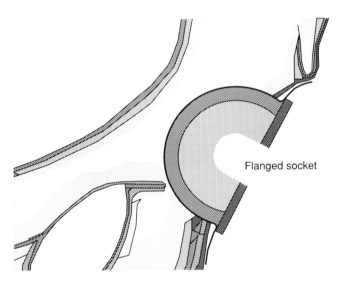

**Figure 10.12**  A flanged socket is introduced that engages with the mesh flap on the periphery and traps it so the complex is 'one-piece'.

Defects or weaknesses in the femur have to be recognized and the new stem must take account of these. Simple endosteal cavitation can be filled with cement and a stem of longer type is passed that bypasses the defect by two stem diameters (Figure 10.14a, b). The tubulation of the femur must be respected and occasional resort is made to endosteal grafting as reported by Gie et al.[11].

Resort can be made to using a mesh reinforcement of a weakened femur to enhance cement stabilization. The mesh is rolled up into a tube shape and placed in the weakened femur (Figure 10.15

a, b, c, d.) The mesh tube acts as a restraint to the cement when the stem is pushed into mesh–cement complex. This method is occasionally of use if the metaphysis of the femur is weakened over a considerable area (Figures 10.15 e, f, g, h, j). When the femur has been prepared the trial stem is inserted to ensure the fit. The Betadine impregnated swab is removed from the acetabulum and the definitive cup is inserted. The trial stem is inserted to test for stability and cemented in situ if satisfactory. The trochanter is re-attached and mobilization allowed when the general condition permits.

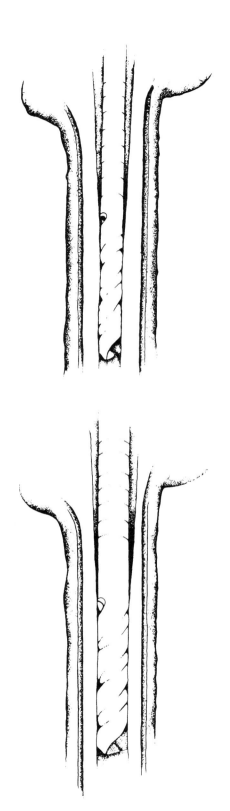

(a)

(b)

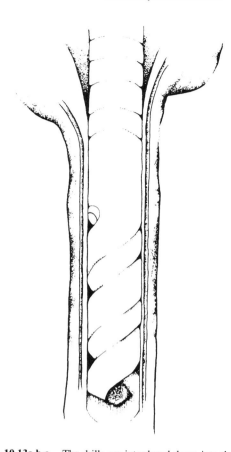

(c)

**Figure 10.13a,b,c,** The drills are introduced down into the cement mantle to reduce the thickness of the mantle. The girth of the drills gradually increases and it is not feasible to pass the drill down to its full extent because the drill is stopped by jamming. It is vital not to apply too much torque to prevent fracture of the shaft of femur.

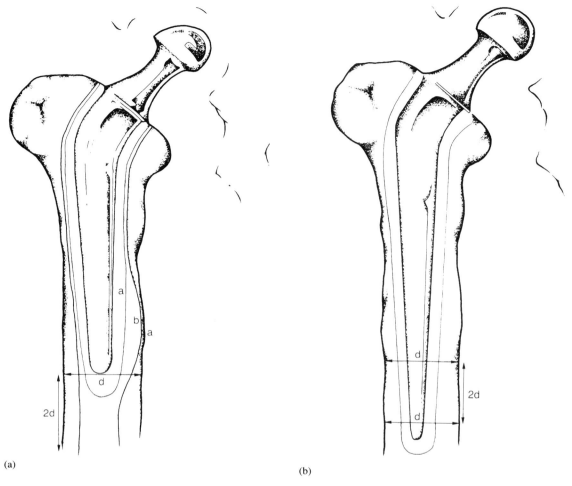

(a)

(b)

**Figure 10.14a,b,** T.M. aged 68. Bilateral THA 16 years prior to radiographs (Figure 10.14a) shown. Severe endosteal bone lysis is shown at Gruen zone 5. The revision must bypass this weakened area by at least two diameters as shown in diagram (Figure 10.14b).

## Illustrative cases

### Direct exchange revision (der)

T.M. aged 68 had undergone bilateral total hip arthroplasty 16 years before for generalized osteoarthrosis. He had been aware for a period of 15 months that walking had gradually become more difficult and he had had to resort to walking aids. The radiographs (Figure 10.16) showed migration of the cup and subsidence of the stem. Endosteal bone lysis is shown in Gruen zone 5 (see Figure 10.2a). and this is shown in the diagram 10.14a at area a.

Direct exchange revision must take account of this weakened bone in the femur at zone b, and a long-stemmed prosthesis is used to by-pass the zone of the weakness by at least two diameters of the shaft of femur below the defect (Figures 10.14b, 10.16a, b).

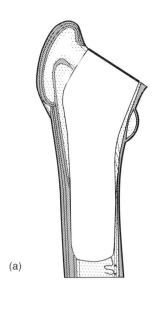

(a)

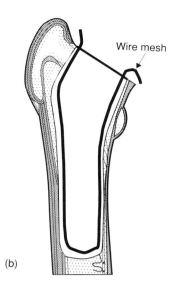

Wire mesh

(b)

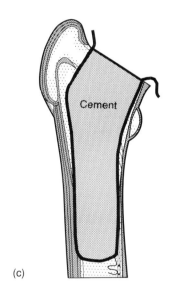

Cement

(c)

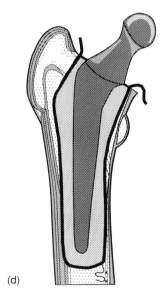

(d)

**Figure 10.15** a, A femur that is weakened by endosteal cavitation but still has an intact tubulation. b, A tube of mesh is inserted but the funnel of mesh is allowed to extend above, so that a flap overlaps the metaphyseal end. c, The mesh funnel is filled with cement. d, The stem of the prosthesis is introduced and a one-piece bone-mesh-cement complex is maintained by the interference overlap of the mesh with the neck of the femur. e, M.T. 6 years after Left Total Hip Arthroplasty showing demarcation in all Gruen zones and subsidence. Radiograph 18.07.84. f, M.T. 3 weeks after revision arthroplasty that had unfortunately been accompanied by a spiral fracture of the femur that had been reduced and fixed by wire encerclage. Radiograph 30.07.84. g, M.T. 3 years after revision total hip arthroplasty, the stem has susbsided down the shaft of femur. Radiograph 15.07.87. The patient has had a conventional primary T.H.A. on the right side which is asymptomatic. h, M.T. 5 months after revision of the left total hip where mesh tubulation was used to act as a constraint in a weakened femur. Radiograph 06.07.88. i, M.T. 7 years after direct exchange revision of the left hip with mesh tubular reinforcement of the femur. Satisfactory appearances clinically and radiologically. Radiograph 17.02.95.

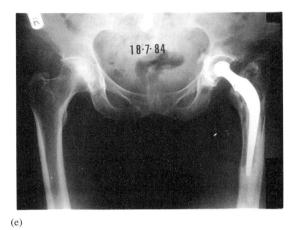

(e)

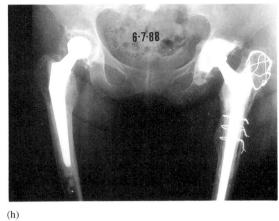

(h)

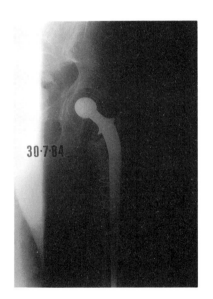

(f)

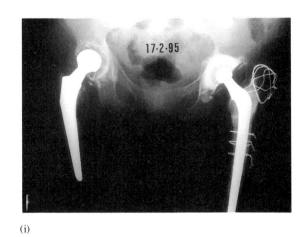

(i)

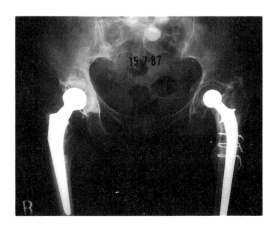

(g)

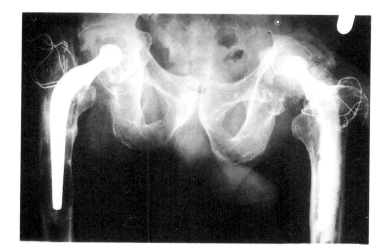

(a)

**Figure 10.16** a, Radiographs of T.M. prior to der. There is severe endosteal osteolysis and scalloping of the cortex. There is severe weakening of the femur at Gruen zone 4 which must be bypassed. b, Revision of the loose stem must use a long stem to bypass the weakened area.

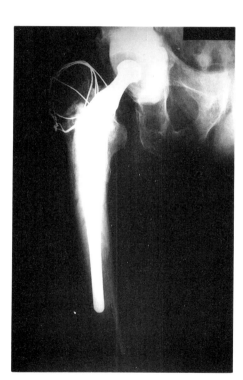

(b)

### Direct exchange revision (der)

This 54-year-old man had injured the left hip in a motorcycle accident and had undergone a McKee–Farrar total hip arthroplasty 12 years before presentation in 1984. The hip arthroplasty was clinically and radiologically loose. (Figure 10.17a). The patient's general condition, the local joint appearances and history suggested an aseptic loosening. The preoperative diagnosis was confirmed by the findings at exploration and the local appearance of the joint tissues, being suggestive of aseptic loosening due to poor cementation; the granulation was grey and fibrotic. A direct exchange revision with adequate cementation is shown in Figure 10.17b. The leg lengths have been equalized. The patient is still well 10 years after the der.

### Interval revision

P.R. female aged 56 years suffering from rheumatoid arthritis (Figure 10.18a) undergoes a right total hip replacement that is initially successful (Figure 10.18b) but after a period of 24 months it was found to be clinically and radiologically loose (Figure 10.18c). At exploration the bone was extremely friable and it was decided to leave the hip as a pseuadarthrosis (Figure 10.18d). After a period of 15 months the bone had recovered sufficiently to permit an interval revision (Figure 10.18e).

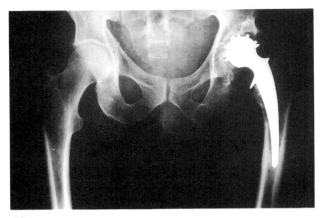

(a)

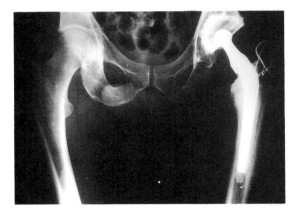

(b)

**Figure 10.17**   a, A Mckee–Farrar total hip arthroplasty that had collapsed into varus, possibly because the diamond-shaped stem of this prosthesis is unfavourable for long-term fixation because the sharp edge cuts the cement. b, Revision with a conforming stem and an adequate cement mantle has resulted in good long-term fixation, no change at 12 years plus.

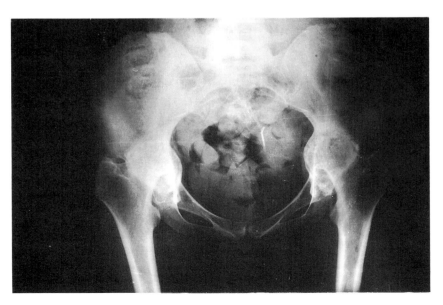

(a)

**Figure 10.18**   a, A 56 year-old female with rheumatoid arthritis has bilateral hip problems with a protrusio acetabulae.

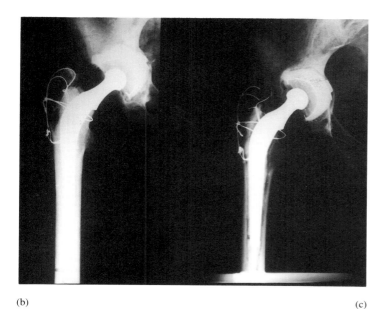

(b)                                                          (c)

b, A total hip replacement is initially successful. c, 24 months later
demarcation of the components is suggestive of septic loosening.

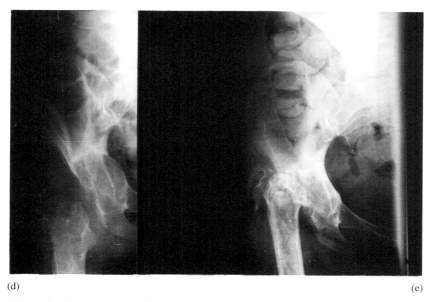

(d)                                                          (e)

d, At exploration there was obvious infection and the bone was friable — all components
removed and pseudarthrosis established. e, 15 months later the bone features have improved
and this was suitable for an internal revision. Postoperative X-rays not shown. (Mr Victor
Burton's case.)

# References

1. De Lee, J. G. and Charnley, J. (1976) Radiological demarcation of cemented sockets in total hip replacement. *Clin. Orthop.*, **121**, 20.
2. Lidwell, O.M. (1982) Effect of ultra-clean air in operating rooms on deep sepsis in the joint after total hip or knee replacement: A randomised study. *Br. Med. J.*, **285**, 10.
3. Charnley, J. (1972) Postoperative infection after total hip replacement with special reference to air contamination in the operating room. *Clin. Orthop.*, **87**, 167.
4. Wilson, P.D. Jr, Agliette, P. and Salvati, E.A. (1974) Subacute sepsis of the hip treated by antibiotics and cemented prosthesis. *J. Bone Joint Surg.*, **56A**, 879.
5. Dupont, J.A. and Lumsden, R.A. (1975) Significance of operative cultures in total joint replacement: *J. Bone Joint Surg.*, **57A**, 138.
6. Williams, E.D., Tregonning, R.H. and Huxley, P.J. (1977) 99 Tm diphosphonate scanning as an aid to diagnosis of infection in patients with a painful total hip prosthesis. *Br.J. Radiol.*, **50**, 582.
7. Williamson, D.R. et al. (1979) Radionuclide bone imaging as a means of differentiating, loosening and infection in patients with a painful total hip prosthesis. *Radiology*, **133**, 723.
8. Lautenbach, E.E.G. and Weber, F.A. (1980) Total hip replacement after chronic hip infection (Proceedings of the South African Orthopaedics Association). *J. Bone Joint Surg.*, **62B**, 282–3.
9. Stuhmer, G. and Weber, B.G. (1978) Die neue Rotation shuftendo-prosthesis nach dem Baukastenprinzp. *System Weber Z. Orthop.*, **116**, 282.
10. Gruen, T.A., McNieve, G.M. and Amstutz, H.G. (1979) Modes of failure of cemented stem type femoral components. A radiological analysis of loosening. *Clin. Orth.*, **141**, 17–27.
11. Gie, G., Linder, L., Ling, R.S.M. et al. (1993) Impaction cancellous allografts and cement for revision total hip arthroplasty. *J.Bone Joint Surg.*, **75B**, 14–21.
12. D'Antonio, J.A., Copello, W.N., Borden, L.S. et al. (1989) Classification and management of acetabular abnormalities in T.H.A. *C.O.R.R.* **243**, 126–137.

# 11

# Cementless femoral revision

Timothy M. Bull and Richard N. Villar

## Why go cementless?

Revision of total hip arthroplasty (THA) is, for many orthopaedic surgeons, becoming a commonplace procedure. Modern prostheses have an anticipated lifespan of around fifteen years or less, especially in young, active patients. Polymethylmethacrylate (PMMA) cement has been shown to fatigue under cyclical loading and its mechanical properties change with time. As more, and younger, patients undergo primary THA, the prospect of multiple revision procedures looms and now revision surgery must try to emulate the success of the primary operation.

Early revision surgeons expected the results of cemented implants to be comparable to primary total hip replacement, but they were soon to be disappointed. The results of cemented revision THA began to appear in the literature in the mid 1980s and showed early failure of the femoral component, in between 20–44% of cases[1–3]. Techniques were developed that improved the longevity of cemented prostheses, including the use of longer stems[4]; though there appears to be a high rate of intra-operative complications with these implants. Harris and co-workers[5] (1988) provided some hope, that by improving the cementing technique the early failure rate could be reduced considerably. Their regime for cementation included femoral washing, a distal cement plug, use of a cement gun and pressurization. All these things are standard practice now for the majority of hip surgeons. At an average follow-up of 74 months, they reported a radiographic loosening rate of 9%, with a further 2% possibly loose. However, the results still did not approach those of primary THA using similar cementing techniques. It is now well recognized that for cement to 'bond' to bone, there must be interlocking of the cement with an irregular bone surface, both macro- and microscopically. Cement has either a very weak or no true molecular bond to bone and does not act like a glue, simply a filler or grout. Aseptic loosening of THA often results in loss of bone stock and the normal trabecular pattern especially in the femur. The resultant surface of bone following removal of the implant, cement, and any membrane, is sclerotic and smooth, with no trabeculae or crevices for cement interdigitation to occur at any level. This fact was investigated by Dohmae and colleagues[6], who showed that the shear strength of the bone–cement interface decreased to 20.6% after a single revision and 6.8% following a second revision procedure, when compared to a primary THA. Cemented revision of acetabular components did not fare any better with early failure rates of 7–34%[1,7]. For these reasons many orthopaedic surgeons started to look for an alternative to cement for revision THA and many cementless designs of prosthesis have evolved for both primary and revision procedures (Figure 11.1). A rationale for the use of cementless designs for revision THA was presented by Hungerford and Jones in 1988[8].

## Indications and planning

There are numerous indications for contemplating revision of a THA, but the most common is painful aseptic loosening. Infection leads to pain and/or loosening, but presents more serious problems

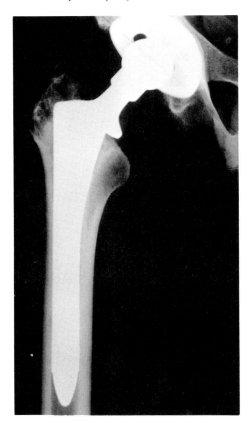

**Figure 11.1** Uncemented revision THA (courtesy of Smith and Nephew–Richards).

when it comes to revision. Other factors such as progressive bone loss with or without femoral stress fracture, deformation or impending prosthesis fracture and recurrent subluxation or dislocation all present relative indications for revision of one or both components. Fractures of the femur or the prostheses must be treated on their own merits. Revision is not always necessary if they cause minimal or no symptoms. Femoral fractures around prostheses can often be treated conservatively or by a lesser procedure such as cerclage wires, Partridge bands or the Mennen plate (CMV).

The potential risks and benefits must be assessed for each patient, particularly if there are serious medical problems coexisting. Revision THA is always a major undertaking, with associated morbidity and mortality, and therefore should not be offered lightly. In respect of the potential complications there is a strong argument for revision hip surgery to be carried out in specific centres, by

surgeons with a special interest in this field. Occasional revision surgeons may not have the resources or the ancillary services available to cope with the complications or rehabilitate the patients after surgery. The patient's fitness for surgery must be assessed and appropriate referral to other specialists made, where necessary, to ensure the patient has every chance of a good outcome.

With revision hip surgery, probably more so than any other form of orthopaedic operation, preoperative planning is essential. The first step is to determine if pain is actually due to a problem within the hip or from another source, e.g. lumbar spine. Single photon emission computerized tomography (SPECT) may play an important role in this respect in the future[9]. MRI scans may be indicated where lumbar spine pathology is suspected of contributing to symptoms. It is important to detect the presence of infection, as many surgeons feel a two-stage procedure is justified when infection is proven. No method of investigation is reliably accurate for detecting infection, apart from intraoperative culture. Gallium scans, hip aspiration and intraoperative Gram stains, when looked at by Kraemer et al.[10], demonstrated low sensitivity compared to culture of specimens taken at surgery. When all this has been completed and a firm decision to revise the THA has been reached, thorough radiographic investigation is the next step. Radiographs will give some indication of bone quality and any deficiencies. For large areas of bone loss (Figure 11.2), sufficient bone graft must be available whether considering the use of autograft, allograft or a combination of these two. The use of bulk allografts or morsellized donor bone should be discussed with the patient prior to surgery, as well as the usual requirement of blood transfusion to ensure they do not have any objection to its use. Leg length discrepancy is difficult to correct accurately during surgery, particularly where there is considerable bone loss and this should also be discussed with the patients to avoid disappointment and litigation.

## Radiography

Radiographs of the pelvis and femur can confirm which components are likely to be loose and allow identification of the implants where case notes are missing or there are inadequate operation records. If only one component is loose then a matching prosthesis should be available, or at the very least, femoral heads or acetabular components of the

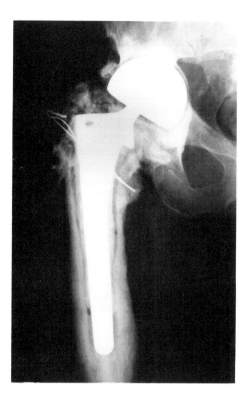

**Figure 11.2** Radiograph showing massive femoral bone loss with failure of cemented primary THA.

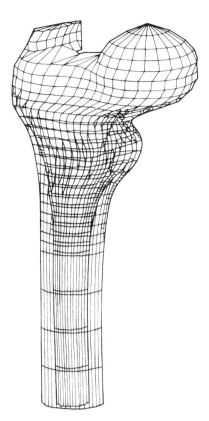

**Figure 11.3** 3D reconstruction of a femur determined from 26 specimens (Clin. Orthop., 1988, **235**, 27).

same diameter as the pre-existing implant. Computerized tomography (CT) is especially useful for deficiences of the acetabulum. Radiographs of the whole length of the femur will show the extent of any cement mantle and also how loose it may be. Appropriate instruments for cement removal can be made available or a plan to 'window' the femur made pre-operatively[11]. If the surgeon chooses to use a long-stem revision prosthesis, femoral bowing is the factor most likely to cause intraoperative complications. This can be considered using full length radiographs. Standardized radiographs can be used to generate three-dimensional computer images of the femur (Figure 11.3) and custom-made implants can then be manufactured.

## The procedure

In all operations meticulous precautions must be taken to avoid introducing infection into an aseptically loose hip arthroplasty. Clean air, laminar flow operating theatres or body exhaust suites must be in use. Prophylactic antibiotics are mandatory, but may be given after appropriate microbiological samples have been taken during the procedure. The approach used for revision THA must ultimately be decided by the individual surgeon. A posterior approach with trochanteric osteotomy allows excellent access to the femoral canal for cement removal, but this has been associated with a high complication rate. Trochanteric osteotomy is responsible for many of the complications, even in primary THA, and should be reserved for exceptional circumstances only[12,13]. Fenestration or splitting of the femur can usually be planned prior to surgery and appropriate meshes, strut allografts and cerclage wires should be available to repair the defects. The pre-existing scar should be incorporated into any approach wherever possible to avoid avascular areas of skin and problems with wound healing. The approach that each individual surgeon is most experienced using is usually the best approach.

Cement removal remains the most time-consuming feature of revision THA and can lead to catastrophe if not meticulously carried out. Where there is infection present all foreign material must be removed including implants, cement, membrane and debris. In any operation where a cementless component is to be introduced, preparation of the femur and/or acetabulum to accept the implant is of paramount importance. All cement and membrane must be removed, allowing any porous coating to impinge on bone in order for bone ingrowth to occur into the implant, thereby achieving a biological fixation. Uncemented primary THA can be very difficult to extract, when good osseointegration has occurred. A range of very narrow-bladed osteotomes and small drills is most useful in this situation.

## Cement extraction

An intact cement mantle can be removed in a variety of ways. Most hospitals have a range of revision cement chisels or osteotomes which require methodical and slow use for the piecemeal removal of cement. The distal cement plug can be drilled and reamed, but this should always be under fluoroscopic control to avoid breaching the cortex. This is especially important when revising curved-stem prostheses or in patients with excessively bowed femurs. The introduction of ultrasonic cement dissolution has revolutionized revision surgery for those who can afford to buy the necessary hardware[14]. A more accessible system utilizes the existing cement mantle[15] a threaded extraction device being used to extract the cement in segments (SEG-CES, Zimmer). This system only works for a conical cement column and has not fully solved the problem of the distal plug.

The acetabulum is often simpler to prepare, but also is more likely to suffer from massive bone loss. Once all the cement is removed a better idea of bony deficiences is gained. Medial and inferior defects can usually be filled with meshes and morselized bone graft, provided there is adequate support around the rim of the cup. Major defects of the anterior or posterior columns, superiorly or laterally can be corrected using bulk grafts. Frozen femoral head allografts are the most available and possibly the easiest to use, although distal femoral allografts are becoming more accessible and useful for major bone loss. They must be securely fixed into the defects and can then be reamed along

with the remainder of the patient's acetabulum to accept a press-fit design cup. Hooten, Engh and Engh[16] reported late migration of uncemented acetabular components into bulk allograft, though this was usually asymptomatic. The degree of migration was related to the area of the cup surface supported by graft, and the use of screw fixation of the cup appears to reduce the migration. Any uncontained graft that is not, therefore, loaded will tend to be resorbed quickly. The results of Pollock and Whiteside[17] show significant acetabular migration in 60% of cases with load-bearing bulk allografts at two years' follow-up. In cases requiring a large amount of graft or where a majority of the graft is expected to be load bearing, it is probably better to consider a cemented acetabular component. Impaction grafting of the femoral side using morsellized bone graft is widely accepted to restore bone stock in the proximal femur, defects can be supported by strut allografts, meshes and cerclage wires. There have been fears that allograft will interfere with the biological fixation of cementless femoral components.

## Choice of prosthesis

The design and manufacture of total hip replacements have recently come under scrutiny because of early failure of many newer prostheses. This is of particular importance in cementless THA designs, where there is no filler material to match up any discrepancies in size or shape, between the prosthesis and the bone surfaces supporting it. All early designs relied on bone ingrowth to occur in order to stabilize the implant, though they were usually a press-fit as well to provide some immediate stability. The implants were designed with large fenestrations or meshes to allow macro-interlock of bone into the structure of the implant and thereby hold it in position. Later designs were coated with titanium beads to provide a greater surface area for bone ingrowth and micro-interlock. This form of porous coating has been extensively investigated, both biochemically and histologically. Bone ingrowth has been shown to occur during the healing phase following the 'injury' of the surgery; thus it only lasts between 6 and 8 weeks; following this stress-induced remodelling commences. Retrieval studies have demonstrated that only a fraction of the porous coated surfaces in both acetabular and femoral components achieves any significant bone ingrowth[18]. Further studies by this same group have shown that osseointegration is even less likely to occur in revision THA[19]. This has been disputed more recently by Sumner et al.[20] who found up to one-third of the void within the porous coating of the Harris–Galante acetabular component filled with bone. It has also been reported that fully porous coated femoral stems can produce proximal bone resorption, which may cause major problems when re-revising them[21, 22].

Micromotion can lead to the formation of fibrous tissue between an implant and bone, thus preventing bone ingrowth. These factors led Poss et al.[23] to question whether porous coating actually conferred any advantages over a simple press-fit design of femoral component. They considered several factors to be important, including initial mechanical stability being afforded by the stem shape. Also, the strength and stiffness of the stem determine the durability and stress remodelling response of the bone and, finally, the surface features of the stem relate to biocompatibility and attachment to bone.

They proposed the 'fit-and-fill' concept for femoral components, where ideally a custom-made implant is used to maximize contact between prosthesis and cortex. A compromise was made to allow manufacture of a range of competitively-priced implants, which maximized contact in the priority areas distal-lateral and proximal-medial (Profile Hip, Dupuy). With any excessively tight-fitting prosthesis, such as this, there is a significant risk of fracture of the femur intraoperatively. Other designs have attempted to create a prosthesis that resembles the normal anatomy of the proximal femur, with a range of sizes to accommodate the majority of patients. Unfortunately, these designs do not match every patient's 'normal' anatomy, more so when there are large bony defects. Another type of hip, the Kent Hip (Biomet), has multiple screwholes to allow interlocking similar to that of intra-medullary nails. This allows femoral fractures around prostheses to be fixed while revising the stem.

Titanium is the material of choice for cementless THA femoral components at this time, as it has a Young's modulus closer to that of bone (approximately half that of cobalt–chrome). It also has been shown to allow bone to grow up to the implant surface and may even have a chemical bond to bone itself. Newer materials, such as carbon-fibre, can be manufactured to have a modulus very close to that of bone and long-term studies are eagerly awaited. The stiffness of any implant, whatever the material it is made of, increases with the diameter, which is a major drawback for cementless THA especially in older patients due to the natural tendency of long bones to expand and undergo cortical atrophy with advancing age.

Cementless acetabular designs have followed two main paths. The hemispherical, press-fit porous coated types, with or without additional screw fixation, have stood the test of time. They readily accommodate placement of bone graft, but for favourable incorporation of bone graft, they require rigid fixation and intimate apposition of the graft to living bone. The alternative screw-in sockets often failed early due to point loading of the threads and even in animal experiments proved unreliable[24]. For revision purposes they were found to be very difficult to use, particularly for larger bony defects as they rely on an interference fit and had a higher failure rate[25].

Hydroxyapatite (HA) ceramic, like polymethylmethacrylate before it, has been used in dentistry for many years. Its potential for use in orthopaedic implants was reported by Lemons in 1988[26]. It forms a strong bond to bone, is osteoconductive when used on porous coated implants and the porosity of its ceramic structure can be varied to allow bony ingrowth into the ceramic itself. With plasma coating a reliable method exists for bonding HA to implants. The chemical composition of the HA and the ceramic structure can be closely controlled and reproduced. More and more cementless THA, both primary and revision, are utilizing HA coatings with very promising short-term results.

## Complications of cementless revision THA

As with any operation there are general complications related to coexisting disease, general anaesthesia, immobility and the stress response to surgical injury. Precautions to prevent these have been mentioned elsewhere, particularly ensuring the patient's fitness prior to embarking on surgery. Antibiotic prophylaxis and attention to asepsis are mandatory. Thromboembolic prophylaxis should also be mandatory, unless there is some specific contraindication.

There are also complications related to revision hip arthroplasty. Vascular injury can occur during any phase of THA. The external iliac artery is particularly at risk, as it may be kinked or compressed while positioning the patient or damaged while preparing the acetabulum. The iliac vessels are most at risk in patients with pre-existing atherosclerosis, but in revision THA they may be tethered by scar tissue or shortened by contracture[27]. Neurological damage can occur at any stage of THA as well.

Positioning to avoid pressure on sciatic, lateral popliteal and the ulnar nerve is important. Damage can occur during the surgical exploration, due to retraction, when dislocating or relocating the prosthesis, during extraction of implants and/or cement, when re-implanting a prosthesis or when wiring femoral fractures, allografts and osteotomies. It should not be forgotten that neurological injury can also occur when the patient is in the recovery area or on the ward if pressure areas are not protected. Heterotopic bone formation is common after THA, but the incidence after trochanteric osteotomy was reported by Duck and Mylod[28] to be 80%. They also reported a decreased range of motion where heterotopic calcification is severe. The incidence of dislocation following revision THA was reported by Williams et al.[29] to be 20%, compared to 0.6% for primary THA. Intraoperative femoral fracture can be a challenging experience to deal with. In the series of 185 revision THAs reported by Morrey and Kavanagh[30], 3% of cemented revision THA and 18% of uncemented revision THA suffered this complication, leading to 4 failures subsequently. This often requires wide exposure of the femur, stripping of soft tissue and the insertion of allograft or some fixation device, thus increasing the risk of sepsis and wound problems. Another series by Christensen et al.[31] showed an incidence of 6.3% femoral fractures, all of which healed but only 60% of these regained satisfactory function. Femoral shaft perforation can occur during cement extraction and femoral reaming. This creates a stress riser and can lead to subsequent fracture. Animal studies have shown that it is preferable to treat these when they occur to prevent later problems[32]. Deep infection rates following revision of aseptically loose THA have been reported as 1.84%[33] when using prophylactic antibiotics and ultra-clean air laminar flow theatres, compared to 0.06% for primary THA under the same conditions. Trochanteric osteotomy has a non-union rate of 13.1% following its use in revision THA[34].

There are some complications more likely to occur following cementless femoral revision THA. Femoral fracture has already been mentioned, the incidence being 6 times higher in cementless revision THA. Thigh pain has proved to be a particular problem in cementless primary and revision

femoral components with an incidence as high as 33% in some series[35]. They also noted 58% of patients had a residual limp, far more than would be expected in a cemented THA series. Fortunately in most series the incidence of thigh pain is less than 10% and usually not disabling. One interesting paper by Barrack et al.[36] reported 6 patients undergoing revision of cementless femoral stems for intractable thigh pain, where secure biological fixation was found at surgery, rendering extraction very difficult. This makes any understanding of the aetiology of thigh pain more difficult to grasp. Early migration of uncemented revision femoral components is a common finding, 15.4% in the series of Engh, Glassman and Suthers[37], but is often asymptomatic. It has, however, been associated with a poorer clinical outcome, even in primary THA, when 3mm or more[35]. HA coating appears to stop the migration of femoral components[38] and may reduce the incidence of thigh pain.

## Does cementless revision THA work?

Short-term reports have shown cementless THA to be a reliable method, with good evidence for osseointegration. Hedley, Gruen and Ruoff[39] reported their series of 61 cementless revisions with a mean follow-up of 20.7 months. Their results showed a 5% re-revision rate, but more than 90% good or excellent results. Gustilo and Pasternak[40] in the same year presented their series of 57 patients, at an average 2.8 years' follow-up and a re-revision rate of 4%. Engh, Glassman and Suthers[37] reported the results of 166 cementless revisions at an average 4.4 years' follow-up. They reported a 1.2% (2/166) overall femoral failure rate with 15.4% incidence of femoral migration on radiographs for proximal porous coated only designs and a 1% incidence of instability for more extensively porous coated prostheses. The acetabular side appeared to be better for hemisherical, porous coated cups, 95–97% had a stable fixation. In their series the screw thread components loosened or migrated in more than 40% of cases. The overall re-revision rate for the acetabular components was 4.8% (8/166).

Longer-term series are now appearing in the literature and are confirming the efficacy of using uncemented systems for revision THA. Lawrence, Engh and Macalino[41] reported a series of 174 revision THAs in 160 patients with a mean follow-up of 7.4 years (range 5–11 years). Their results show a 5.7% re-revision rate, with evidence of loosening radiographically in another 1.1%. A subsequent paper by Lawrence et al.[42], with a mean follow-up of 9 years reported a femoral re-revision rate of 10% and acetabular re-revision rate of 7%, with physician-defined success rate of 83% and a patient satisfaction of 93%. Head et al.[43] reported their results of uncemented revision THA and cortical onlay strut allografts for structurally deficient femurs. They show grafts united in 98% of their patients and had evidence of revascularization. They also reported 3.4% (6/174) re-revision rate for femoral failure. Kolstad's series[44] looked at revision of THA because of femoral fracture. They compared the results of using conventional long-stem implants with the Wagner uncemented system. They report all fractures healed, but 7/14 conventional implants loosened and all 9 Wagners in their series showed no signs of loosening.

The use of hydroxyapatite coatings on orthopaedic implants is still very much in its infancy. A few series looking at early stability and short-term results are available. Drucker et al.[45] presented their results at an average 10.4 months in both primary and revision THA. The patients appeared to have little or no pain in 96% and could walk without aids in 95%. No patient reviewed radiographically after one year showed any signs of loosening or migration. Geesink[46] reported no signs of loosening either clinically or radiographically until at least 6 years postoperatively, where a HA-coated prosthesis was used.

## Summary

The rationale for the use of cementless revision THA evolved out of the disappointing results of revision surgery using cement. Since the mid 1980s many different types of uncemented prostheses have been developed, though most are very similar in design and construction. The cementless THA lends itself well to bone grafting procedures, especially on the acetabular side. There are more complications associated with the use of cementless THA, most serious being intraoperative fractures, migration of components and subsequent difficulty with re-revising well osseointegrated implants. The results show that while cementless revision THA still does not compare with properly cemented primary THA, it compares favourably with cemented revision THA. With the advent of HA coating things should continue to improve.

## References

1. Kavanagh, B.F., Ilstrup, D.M. and Fitzgerald, R.H. Jr (1985) Revision of total hip arthroplasty. *J. Bone Joint Surg.*, **67A**, 517–526.
2. Pellici, P.M., Wilson, P.D. and Sledge, C.B. (1985) Long term results of revision total hip replacement: a follow up report. *J. Bone Joint Surg.*, **67A**, 513–516.
3. Stromberg, C.N., Herberts, P. and Ahnfelt, L. (1988) Revision total hip replacement in patients younger than 55 years: clinical and radiological results after 4 years. *J. Arthroplasty*, **3**, 47–52.
4. Turner, R.H., Mattingly, D.A. and Scheller, A. (1987) Femoral revision total hip arthroplasty using long stem femoral components. *J. Arthroplasty*, **2**, 247–251.
5. Rubash, H.E. and Harris, W.H. (1988) Revision of non-septic, loose, cemented femoral components using modern cementing techniques. *J. Arthroplasty*, **3**, 241–248.
6. Dohmae, Y., Bechtold, J.E. and Sherman, R.E. (1988) Reduction in cement-bone interface shear strength between primary and revision arthroplasty. *Clin. Orthop.*, **236**, 214–220.
7. Callaghan, J.T., Salvati, E.A., Pellicci, P. et al. (1985) Results of revision for mechanical failure after cemented total hip replacement. *J. Bone Surg.*, **67A**, 1074–1085.
8. Hungerford, D.S. and Jones, L.C. (1988) The rationale of cementless revision of cemented arthroplasty failures. *Clin. Orthop.*, **235**, 12–24.
9. Ryan, P.J., Evans, P.A., Gibson, T. and Fogelman, I. (1992) Chronic low back pain: comparison of bone SPECT with radiography and CT. *Radiology*, **182**, 849–854.
10. Kraemer, W.J., Saplys, R., Waddell, J.P. and Morton, J. (1993) Bone scan, gallium scan and hip aspiration in the diagnosis of infected total hip arthroplasty. *J. Arthroplasty*, **8**, 611–616.
11. Klein, A.H. and Rubash, H.E. (1993) Femoral windows in revision total hip arthroplasty. *Clin. Orthop.*, **291**, 164–170.
12. Frankel, A., Booth, R.E. Jr, Balderston, R.A. et al. (1993) Complications of trochanteric osteotomy: long term implications. *Clin. Orthop.*, **288**, 209–213.
13. Glassman, A.H. (1992) Complications of trochanteric osteotomy. *Orthop. Clin. North Am.*, **23**(2), 321–333.
14. Klapper, R.C., Caillouette, J.T., Callaghan, J.J. and Hozack, W.J. (1992) Ultrasonic technology in revision joint arthroplasty. *Clin. Orthop.*, **285**, 147–154.
15. Ekelund, A.L. (1992) Cement removal in revision hip arthroplasty: experience with bone cement added to the cavity in 20 cases. *Acta Orthop. Scand.*, **63**, 549–551.
16. Hooten, J.P. Jr, Engh, C.A. Jr and Engh, C.A. (1994) Failure of structural acetabular allografts in cementless revision hip arthroplasty. *J. Bone Joint Surg.*, **76B**, 419–422.
17. Pollock, F.H. and Whiteside, L.A. (1992) The fate of massive allografts in total hip acetabular revision surgery. *J. Arthroplasty*, **7**, 271–276.
18. Haddad, R.J. Jr, Cook, S.D. and Thomas, K.A. (1987) Biological fixation of porous coated implants. *J. Bone Joint Surg.*, **69A**, 1459–1466.
19. Cook, S.D., Barrack, R.L., Thomas, K.A. and Haddad, R.J. Jr (1991) Tissue growth into porous primary and revision femoral stems. *J. Arthroplasty*, **6**, Suppl. 37–46.
20. Sumner, D.R., Jasty, M., Jacobs, J.J. et al. (1993) Histology of porous coated acetabular components: 25 cementless cups retrieved after arthroplasty. *Acta Orthop. Scand.* 1993; 64: 619–26.
21. Brown, J.W. and Ring, P.A. (1985) Osteolytic changes in the upper femoral shaft following porous coated hip replacement. *J. Bone Joint Surg.*, **67B**, 218–221.

22. Turner, T.M., Sumner, D.R., Urban, Rivero, D.P. et al. (1986) A Comparative Study of porous coatings in a weight bearing total hip arthroplasty model. *J. Bone Joint Surg.*, **68A**, 1396–1409.

23. Poss, R., Walker, P., Spector, M. et al. (1988) Strategies for improving fixation of femoral components in total hip arthroplasty. *Clin. Orthop.*, **235**, 181–194.

24. Tooke, S.M., Nugent, P.J., Chotivichit, A. et al. (1988) Comparison of in vivo cementless acetabular fixation. *Clin. Orthop.*, **235**, 253–260.

25. More, R.C., Amstutz, H.C., Kabo, J.M. et al. (1992) Acetabular reconstruction with a threaded prosthesis for failed total hip arthroplasty. *Clin. Orthop.*, **282**, 114–122.

26. Lemons, J.E. (1988) Hydroxyapatite coatings. *Clin. Orthop.*, **235**, 220–223.

27. Matos, M.H., Amstutz, H.C. and Machleder, H.I. (1979) Ischaemia of the lower extremity after total hip replacement. *J. Bone Joint Surg.*, **61A**, 24–27.

28. Duck, H.J. and Mylod, A.G. Jr (1992). Heterotopic bone in hip arthroplasties: cemented versus non-cemented. *Clin. Orthop.*, **282**, 145–153.

29. Williams, J.F., Gottesman, M.J. and Mallory, T.H. (1982) Dislocation after total hip arthroplasty: treatment with an above knee hip spica cast. *Clin. Orthop.*, **171**, 53–58.

30. Morrey, B.F. and Kavanagh, B.F. (1992) Complications of revision of the femoral component of total hip arthroplasty: comparison between cemented and uncemented techniques. *J. Arthroplasty*, **7**, 71–79.

31. Christensen, C.M., Seger, B.M. and Schultz, R.B. (1989) Management of intra-operative femur fractures associated with revision hip arthroplasty. *Clin. Orthop.*, **248**, 177–180.

32. Doyle, J., Procter, P. and Moloney, M.A. (1990) Femoral shaft perforation at arthroplasty: to treat or not to treat? *Arch. Orthop. Trauma Surg.*, **109**, 217–220.

33. Fitzgerald, R.H. Jr. (1992) Total hip arthroplasty sepsis: prevention and diagnosis. *Orthop. Clin. North Am.*, **23**(2), 259–264.

34. Amstutz, H.C., Ma, S.M., Jinnah, R.H. and Mai, L. (1982) Revision of aseptic, loose total hip arthroplasty. *Clin. Orthop.* **170**, 21–33.

35. Maric, Z. and Karpman, R.R. (1992) Early failure of non-cemented porous coated anatomic total hip arthroplasty. *Clin. Orthop.*, **278**, 116–120.

36. Barrack, R.L., Jasty, M., Bragdon, C. et al. (1992) Thigh pain despite bone ingrowth into uncemented femoral stems. *J. Bone Joint Surg.*, **74B**, 507–510.

37. Engh, C.A., Glassman, A.H. and Suthers, K.E. (1990). The case for porous-coated hip implants: the femoral side. *Clin. Orthop.*, **261**, 63–81.

38. Karrholm, J., Malchau, H., Snorrason, F. and Herberts, P. (1994) Micromotion of femoral stems in total hip arthroplasty. *J. Bone Joint Surg.*, **76A**, 1692–1705.

39. Hedley, A.K., Gruen, T.A. and Ruoff, O.P. (1988) Revision of failed total hip arthroplasties with uncemented porous-coated anatomic components. *Clin. Orthop.*, **235**, 75–90.

40. Gustilo, R.B. and Pasternak, H.S. (1988) Revision total hip arthroplasty with titanium ingrowth prosthesis and bone grafting for failed cemented femoral component loosening. *Clin. Orthop.*, **235**, 111–119.

41. Lawrence, J.M., Engh, C.A. and Macalino, G.E. (1993) Revision total hip arthroplasty: long term results without cement. *Orthop. Clin. North Am.*, **24**(4), 635–644.

42. Lawrence, J.M., Engh, C.A., Macalino, G.E. and Lauro, G.R. (1994) Outcome of revision hip arthroplasty done without cement. *J. Bone Joint Surg.*, **76A**, 965–973.

43. Head, W.C., Wagner, R.A., Emerson, R.H. Jr and Malinin, T.I. (1994) Revision total hip arthroplasty in the deficient femur with a proximal load-bearing prosthesis. *Clin. Orthop.*, **298**, 119–126.

44. Kolstad, K. (1994) Revision total hip replacement after peri-prosthetic femoral fractures: an analysis of 23 cases. *Acta Orthop. Scand.*, **65**, 505–508.

45. Drucker, D.A., Capello, W.N., D'Antonio, J.A. and Hile, L.E. (1991) Works in progress 6: total hip arthroplasty using a hydroxyapatite coated acetabular and femoral component. *Orthop. Rev.*, **20**, 179–185.

46. Geesink, R.G. (1993) Clinical, radiological and human histological experience with hydroxyapatite coatings in orthopaedic surgery. *Acta Orthop. Belgica*, **59**, Suppl. 160–164.

# 12

# Femoral component revision: the rationale for custom design

Chitranjan S. Ranawat, Michael M. Alexiades, Jose A. Rodriguez, Bruce H. Robie and Timothy M. Wright

## Introduction

The uniformly successful clinical outcome following femoral component revision has been difficult to achieve with either cemented or uncemented stems. Older studies of revision surgery have had results which were less than optimal, with a high intraoperative complication rate and a high aseptic loosening rate[1–3, 20, 21]. Because of the unsatisfactory results following cemented femoral revision, uncemented revision total hip arthroplasty has been an area of intense study in recent years.

In uncemented revision arthroplasty it can be difficult to obtain rigid fixation with stability in all three planes of axial, bending, and torsional moments using conventional stems. Factors such as proximal femoral bone loss, altered bone geometry, poor bone quality and blood supply all predispose to inadequate fixation of the femoral component and therefore a less predictable clinical result. This has led to additional interest in the area of custom designed implants, with the hope of achieving a better fit, and thereby an improved, reproducible clinical result.[25]

## Biomechanics

The general biomechanical goals for revision total hip replacement are the same as for most total joint replacements:

1. Establish or re-establish normal kinematics;
2. Provide for appropriate load transfer to the surrounding bone;
3. Assure the long-term performance of the device.

For total hip replacements, the kinematics are modelled as a ball and socket joint. Re-establishment of the normal kinematics demands proper placement of the femoral head in space, which is determined in three dimensions. Appropriate reconstruction requires re-establishment of the height, offset, and anteversion of the femur. Restoration of the height creates adequate soft-tissue tension in the muscles across the hip joint, and restoration of the offset assures the abductor muscle's necessary mechanical advantage to function normally. Failure to restore either the height or the offset can result in increased energy expenditure to achieve the same joint kinematcs. Similarly, reduction in either height or offset can diminish the inherent stability of the construct, increase the joint load, and possibly reduce the long-term performance of the revision total hip replacement.

Restoration of the correct anteversion provides a mechanical balance between the flexors and extensors of the hip. Excessive anteversion reduces the mechanical advantage in the flexors, making flexion more difficult, and increases the mechanical advantage of the extensors, making extension easier. However, too little anteversion has opposite results. Inappropriate anteversion will also increase the risk of dislocation due to inherent limitations of motion in the implant as well as changes in the resting lengths of the muscles around the hip with resulting imbalance.

In complex revision surgery it is often difficult to maintain muscular attachments to the proximal femur. For example, non-union of the greater trochanter can frequently occur, or bony defects in the proximal metaphysis of the femur can require the use of allografts to augment or replace the proximal femur. Loss of the muscular attachment reduces the stability of the hip and may adversely affect the kinematics of the joint. Loss of muscular attachments to the proximal femur also results in changes on the loads on the femur and pelvis, and affect the joint load necessary to establish equilibrium. In addition, loss of muscle attachments results in devascularization of portions of the proximal femur, which affects the potential for bony ingrowth onto uncemented components, and may impair the long-term fixation of the implant.

Long-term load transfer to the femur is a significant problem in revision total hip replacement surgery. Davie et al. determined the maximal load on the femur to be 2.8 times body weight oriented 10–20° laterally from the axis of the femur, and posteriorly 15–25° with respect to the implant[4]. This load, therefore, has a significant vertical component which compresses the implant into the femur. Since vertical load is applied through the head, which is offset from the implant, significant bending loads are applied to the implant. In addition, the posteriorly directed load component also affects load transfer, especially in activities such as stair climbing and getting up from seated positions even though the vertical component of the load is small for such an activity. This posteriorly directed load component applied through the head centre generates a torsional moment along the long axis of the femur and will cause the femoral component to spin within the bone.

Load transfer from the femoral components in revision total hip replacements must consider all three loads: axial, bending and torsional. Transmission of compressive loads can occur in one of two ways: the implant can abut the bone in the direction of the compressive load, or the load can be transferred through a sheer interface. Transferring the compressive load through an abutment can occur through collars, step cuts, or

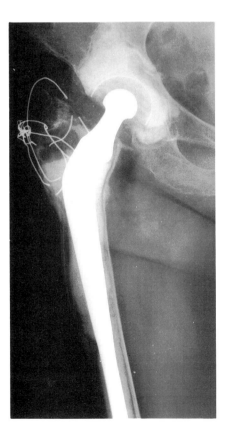

(a)

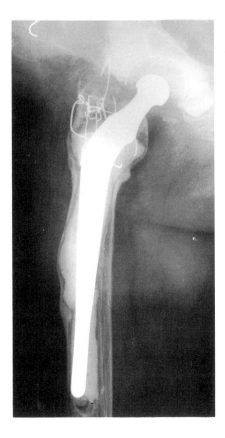

(b)

**Figure 12.1**   a, Anteroposterior and b, lateral views of the right hip in a patient with a loose, subsided femoral stem after two previous revisions. There was metaphysial and diaphysial segmental bone loss, as well as angular deformity of the proximal femur requiring intraoperative corrective osteotomy.

tapers in the implant and the bone. Since patients undergoing revision surgery often have poor proximal bone stock, it may be difficult in off-the-shelf designs to achieve bone apposition where the bone tapers. Similarly with modular designs, orienting the proximal component to a 'best fit' position within the metaphysis remains a compromise in deficient bone stock. The second way to transfer compressive loads is to develop an interface capable of carrying large amounts of shear, such that load transfer can occur in the tubular region of the bone. Two common ways are to use porous coating or a very rough sandblasting on the more distal portions of the femoral component stem. Bending moments can be resisted more easily than compressive loads by using a press-fit cylindrical stem in a canal of appropriate length that will provide stability and long-term load transfer. To ensure stability the length of the stem should be at least two bone diameters.

Transmission of torsional loads is difficult to achieve. Since the torque tends to rotate the implant posteriorly, posterior support in the proximal metaphysis is very helpful, and the geometry of the bone is critical. There should be a medial flare of the proximal metaphysis as the femur extends up into the neck for proximal torsional support to be of any value. In a revision situation, custom design achieves torsional control through intimate contact with available bone.

The long-term performance of revision total hip replacements has not been uniformly good[3,5]. Most of the failures are due to loosening, resulting in either subsidence or retroversion of the stem with respect to the shaft of the femur. For this reason optimization of load transfer and initial fixation have become a primary focus of research.

There are three fundamental approaches to load transfer in this revision situation. One is to attempt to regain proximal load transfer in torsion and

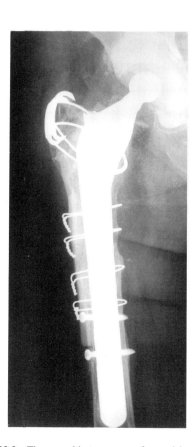
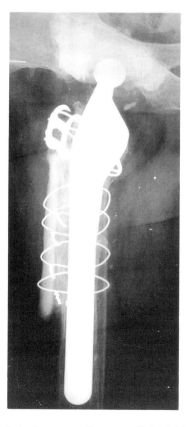

**Figure 12.2** The same hip two years after revision with a custom femoral component which was five-eighths porous-coated, proximal loading, with interlocking screws into an elliptical hole in the stem to allow controlled subsidence. A strut allograft was used as fixation for the diaphyseal osteotomy.

compression, as in a well fit proximally coated stem. Another approach concedes proximal load transfer, and instead transfers the load distally through roughened or porous coated surfaces tightly fitted to the diaphyseal bone. A third option is to seek distal torsional control with proximal axial load transfer using a modular or custom component. Each scenario has its own advantages and disadvantages. Exclusive proximal load transfer in a femur with extensive bone loss risks eventual failure due to lack of bony support with uneven distribution of loads unless an intimate fit of the implant is achieved. Exclusive distal load transfer increases the torsional and bending forces on the implant distally, increasing the risk of implant failure as well as proximal bony resorption.

Femoral stem geometry has also been addressed to determine whether a straight stem or an anatomical (curved) stem design results in better fixation and improved interface motion. Callaghan et al. compared the torsional and axial loads in cadavers utilizing an uncemented, collarless, isthmus filling, straight stem and an uncemented, collarless, anatomical stem[6]. There were no significant differences in the magnitudes of motion of the femoral components with axial loads. There was, however, significantly less motion noted with anatomical stems in response to torsional loads.

The significance of motion in the uncemented component relates to its effect on bone ingrowth. Motion has been shown to be detrimental to bony ingrowth and to enhance fibrous tissue ingrowth[7]. Retrieval studies of uncemented components have found as little as 4% bony ingrowth in what appeared to be well fixed components[8]. Other investigators have revealed that in primary porous coated femoral stems the bone ingrowth is minimal to moderate at most, and in revision cases the percentage of bone ingrowth was even less than in primary femoral stems[9].

## Clinical review

### Cemented revisions

Revision total hip arthroplasty using cement fixation has had variable results with re-revision rates ranging from 5% to 20% within 8 years of surgery[1, 5, 24, 26]. In addition, cement fixation is ill suited to compensate for segmental bone loss in the femoral metaphysis and diaphysis (Figure 12.1). For these reasons uncemented fixation has been pursued by many surgeons as a potentially better option in complex revision surgery.

### Uncemented revisions

The use of uncemented techniques, however, has not provided a uniformly successful reconstruction. With less than 5 years follow-up, re-revision rates have ranged from 6% to 20%, with radiographic presumption of loosening in up to 43% of implants[5, 10, 19, 23]. Unfortunately most of these studies cannot be adequately compared due to incomplete documentation of important factors related to outcome, such as extent of bone loss, bone quality, patient age, and activity level.

Our indications for the use of custom implants for revision hip arthroplasty include major deformity, and bone loss, where standard cemented and uncemented implants inadequately address the anatomical and biomechanical problems of reconstruction. In comparing recent data on complex revision surgery some valuable observations can be made (Table 12.1).

In a review of 174 femoral revisions, Lawrence et al. classified 39 cases as having severely deficient bone stock, requiring a fully coated, long-stemmed device for diaphyseal fixation[11]. In some instances the long straight stem used early in the study perforated the anterior cortex. Eight implants in the severely bone deficient cohort (20%) required re-revision, and one was radiographically unstable.

**Table 12.1  Comparison of revision surgery**

| Author | Implant | # hips | Follow-up time (years) | % type III bone loss | Re-revisions for loosening | Subsidence | Intraop fxs |
|--------|---------|--------|-----------------------|---------------------|---------------------------|------------|-------------|
| Malkani | Custom | 23 | 2–5 | 52 | 0 | 0–6 mm | 8 (35%) |
| Bargar | Custom | 47 | 2–4 | 57 | 1 (2%) | 15% 5–10 mm | 9 (19%) |
| Cameron | Modular | 91 | 2–6 | 68 | 4 (4%) | Not reported | 4 (4%) |
| Head | Calcar replacement | 177 | 2–6 | 54 | 6 (3%) | 5 hips > 1 cm | Not reported |
| Lawrence | AML – fully coated | 39 | 5–9 | 100 | 8 (20%) | 1 hip | Not reported |

**Table 12.2   Classification system for femoral bone loss proposed by Papyrosky et al.[16]**

| Type | Metaphysis | Calcar femorale | Diaphysis |
|------|-----------|-----------------|-----------|
| I | Intact | Partially gone Minor anterior and posterior loss | Intact |
| IIA | Cavitary defect Subtrochanteric region intact | Absent | Intact |
| IIB | Segmental loss of anterolateral portion of subtrochanteric bone | Absent | intact |
| IIC | Medial wall absent to level of diaphysis. Completely non-supportive | Absent | Bone loss which impairs rotational control |

Head et al. have reported on a review of 177 revision total hip arthroplasties in deficient femora with 2–6 year follow-up[12]. In his series 54% of the cases had type III femoral bone loss with extensive metaphyseal and diaphyseal defects. Using long, proximally coated calcar replacement implants they sought axial and rotational stability and ingrowth within the proximal one-third of the stem. All of the cases were reconstructed using cortical strut allografts, usually to augment medial deficiency. In this series 6 hips (3%) required re-revision, and 5 hips had subsidence of greater than 1 cm. Of the revised cases, 2 loosened as a result of supporting the implant on structural allograft, and 2 hips had severe end of stem pain.

Cameron has published his results using a modular titanium implant, seeking distal rotational control, and proximal load transfer[13]. In his series of 91 hips, 68% had significant femoral bone loss requiring the use of a long stemmed component, and intraoperative fractures occurred in 7 cases (8%). Structural allografting was necessary in only 3 hips with this modular design. At 2–6 years of follow-up, four hips (4%) have required re-revision for anterior perforation of the stem, and one had significant end of stem pain with an early solid version of the implant. Of the unrevised cased 23% had mild to moderate thigh pain.

**Custom revisions**

The use of custom implants has been espoused by Bargar et al., who recently reviewed their experience with 47 revision total hip arthroplasties[14, 15]. Type III femoral bone defects were present in 57% of cases, and intraoperative fractures occurred in 19% of cases. At 2–4 years of follow-up, one implant has been revised for loosening. Fifteen per cent of the implants had subsided 5–10 mm with the early collarless design, which utilized only anterior, posterior and medial ingrowth pads. No structural allografts were required for stability.

Malkani et al. have reviewed the Hospital for Special Surgery experience with 23 total hip replacements revised using a custom femoral component[22]. In each case significant bony defects were the reason for choosing a custom design, with 52% of the cases assessed as having a type III bony defect (Table 12.2). Eight hips (35%) had intraoperative fractures of the attenuated metaphysis during implantation. These were treated with cerclage wiring, with no change in the postoperative protocol. The implants were collarless, with the porous surface applied circumferentially to the proximal one-third of the implant. In cases where rotational control was not achievable proximally, additional flutes, porous surface, or interlocking screws were added distally. With this design, the average subsidence at 2–5 years of follow-up was 3 mm (range 0–6 mm). None of the implants have yet required revision and no structural allografting was required. However, 9 hips (41%) had mild, activity related pain.

In the latter three studies the clinical results reported were all equivalent, with Harris hip scores averaging 80–85. However, other issues such as the prevalence of thigh pain and limp, and the actual effect on functional outcome are incompletely addressed. The major problem in comparing these clinical series is the fact that no single classification system is used for describing bone loss.

Implant costs have, in the past, been a concern of hospitals in deciding between implants. Modern CAD-CAM techniques have resulted in a reduction in the manufacturing cost for custom devices[17], and manufacturing costs for modular titanium implants are similar. As a result, custom components and modular components are comparable with regards to cost.

We favour the use of custom implants in cases of significant femoral bone loss. A computerized tomogram can assist in the decision-making process in that femoral bone stock and abnormal geometry can be assessed. This approach allows the surgeon to tailor the implant to the particular situation, while avoiding the use of structural bone grafting for stability. In this way, load transfer to existing bone is optimized, while additional grafting to replenish bone stock remains an option.

In cases where rotational stability cannot be achieved proximally, interlocking screws can be used in an elliptical hole in the stem to allow controlled subsidence and stabilization (Figure 12.2). In addition, porous surface can be applied selectively to areas where stability and ingrowth can be achieved, potentially minimizing proximal bone resorption associated with a stiff, distally fixed implant. In this way the potential negative aspects of interface fretting and corrosion of the modular interfaces can also be avoided[18] (see Table 12.1).

In summary, the use of custom femoral components can optimize load transfer, while compensating for bone loss, and thereby reproduce the geometry and kinematics of the hip. Short-term studies suggest a more predictable clinical course than has been reported for standard, off-the-shelf, cemented and uncemented components. Long-term studies should reveal whether the use of these devices will actually improve the functionality and longevity of these reconstructions.

## References

1. Franzen, H., Mjoberg, B. and Onnerfalt, R. (1992) Early loosening of femoral components after cemented revision. A roentgen stereophotogrammetric study (published erratum appears in *J. Bone Joint Surg., 75B* 169, 1993). *J. Bone Joint Surg., 74B*, 721–724.
2. Gustilo, R.B., Bechtold, J.E., Giachetto, J. and Kyle, R.F. (1989) Rationale, experience, and results of long-stem femoral prostheses. *Clin. Orthop., 249* 159–168.
3. Morrey, B.F. and Kavanagh B.F. (1992) Complications with revision of the femoral component of total hip arthroplasty. Comparison between cemented and uncemented techniques. *J. Arthroplasty, 7*, 71–79.
4. Davy, D.J., Kotzar, G.T., Brown, R.H. et al. (1988) Telemetric force measurements across the hip after total arthroplasty. *J. Bone Joint Surg., 70A*, 45–50.
5. Stromberg, C.N., Herberts, P. and Ahnfelt, L. (1988) Revision total hip arthroplasty in patients younger than 55 years old. Clinical and radiologic results after 4 years. *J. Arthroplasty, 3*, 47–59.
6. Callaghan, J.J., Fulghum, C.S., Glisson, R.R. and Stranne, S.K. (1992) The effect of femoral stem geometry on inter-face motion in uncemented porous-coated total hip prostheses. Comparison of straight stem and curved stem designs. *J. Bone Joint Surg., 74A*, 839–848.
7. Pilliar, R.M., Lee, J.M. and Maniatopoulos. C. (1986) Observations on the effect of movement on bone ingrowth into porous-surfaced implants. *Clin. Orthop., 208*, 108–113.
8. Jasty, M., Bragdon, C.R., Maloney, W.J. et al. (1991) Ingrowth of bone in failed fixation of porous-coated femoral components. *J. Bone Joint Surg., 73A*, 1331–1337.
9. Cook, S.D., Barrack, R.L., Thomas, K.A. and Haddad, Jr, R.J. (1991) Tissue growth into porous primary and revision femoral stems. *J. Arthroplasty, 6*, Suppl. S37–46.
10. Malkani, A.L., Lewallen, D.G., Cabanela, M.E. (1993) Two to five-year follow up of femoral component revisions using an uncemented, proximally-coated chrome cobalt, long-stem prosthesis. Annual Meeting of American Academy of Orthopaedic Surgery February, San Francisco, California USA.
11. Lawrence, J.M., Engh, C.A. and Macalino, G.E. (1993) Revision total hip arthoplasty. *Orthop. Clin. North Am., 124*, 635.
12. Head, W.C., Wagner, R.A., Emerson, R.H., and Malinin, T.J. (1994) Revision total hip arthroplasty in the deficient femur with a proximal load-bearing prosthesis. *Clin. Orthop., 298*, 119–126.
13. Cameron, H.U. (1994) The two- to six-year results with a proximally modular noncemented total hip replacement used in hip revisions. *Clin. Orthop., 298*, 47–53.
14. Barger, W.L. (1989) Shape the implant to the patient. A rationale for the use of custom-fit cementless total hip implants. *Clin. Orthop., 249*; 73–78.
15. Barger, W.L., Murzic, W.J., Taylor, J.K. et al. (1993) Management of bone loss in revision total hip arthroplasty using custom femoral components. *J. Arthroplasty, 8*, 245–252.
16. Paprosky, W., Lawrence, J. and Cameron, H. (1990) Femoral defect classification: Clinical application. *Orthop. Rev., 19* (Suppl. 9) 9.
17. Crawford, H.V., Unwin, P.S. and Walker, P.S. (1992) The CADCAM contribution to customized orthopaedic implant. *Proc. Inst. Mech. Eng. 206*, 43–46.
18. Bobyn, J.D., Tanzer, M., Krygier, J.J. et al. (1994) Concerns with modularity in total hip arthroplasty. *Clin. Orthop., 298*, 27–36.
19. Eskola, A., Santavirta, S.J., Konttinen, Y.T. et al. (1990) Cementless revision of aggressive granulomatous lesions in hip replacements. *J. Bone Joint Surg. 72B*, 212–216.
20. Hedley, A.K., Gruen, T.A. and Ruoff, D.P. (1988) Revision of failed total hip arthroplasties with uncemented porous-coated anatomic components. *Clin. Orthop., 235*, 75–90.
21. Kavanaugh, B.F. and Fitzgerald, Jr., R.H. (1992) Multiple revisions for failed total hip arthroplasty not associated with infection. *J. Bone Joint Surg., 69A*, 1144–1149.
22. Malkani, A.L., Figgie, M.P. and Ranawat, C.S. (1993) Custom femoral components for revision total hip replacement. Annual Meeting of International Society for the Study of Custom Prostheses. October, Amelia Island, Florida USA.
23. Rivero, D.P., Galante, J.O., Kull, L. and Moher, C.G. (1993) Femoral revision: Inadequacy of proximally coated femoral components at average four years follow-up. Annual Meeting of American Academy of Orthopaedic Surgeons, February, San Francisco, CA.
24. Rubash, H.E. and Harris, W.H. (1988) Revision of nonseptic, loose cemented femoral components using modern cement techniques. *J. Arthroplasty, 3*, 241–248.

25. Stulberg, S.D., Stulberg, B.N. and Wixson, R.L. (1989) The rationale, design characteristics, and preliminary results of a primary custom total hip prosthesis. *Clin. Orthop., 249*, 79–96.

26. Turner, R.H., Mattingly, D.A. and Scheller, A. (1987) Femoral revision total hip arthroplasty using a long-stem femoral component. Clinical and radiographic analysis. *J. Arthroplasty, 2*, 247–258.

# 13

# Reconstruction of the acetabulum

Allan E. Gross

Restoration of bone stock on the pelvic side in arthroplasty of the hip is a difficult and controversial area. The spectrum of surgical opinion goes from avoiding the use of bone graft if at all possible[1] to the use of morsellized bone only[2] to the use of complex structural grafts[3].

There is no question that structural grafts on the pelvic side have a guarded prognosis and should be avoided if possible[4]. At the same time there are situations where bulk allograft has to be used, and if used properly can yield acceptable results and restore bone stock for future surgery[4].

It is imperative that the principles of bone grafting be understood and adhered to in order to optimize consults.

Bone grafts are classified into heterografts (bone from another species), allografts (bone from the same species) and autograft (bone taken from one part of the same individual). In the revision situation because of the quantity and quality of bone required allograft is more practical than autograft. There are, however, certain advantages and disadvantages of each.

Autograft has the advantages of not being immunogenic and even more importantly is best for inducing new bone formation in the host. Its disadvantages are the quantity available, the strength, shape and form which cannot duplicate the deficit.

Allografts on the other hand are available in quantity and can be strong and duplicate the deficit. They are, however, immunogenic[5–7] and are not as effective as autografts for inducing new bone formation[5,7,8].

Bone deficits on the pelvic side are classified as follows:

1. *Protrusio*: A contained cavitary defect with the acetabular walls and columns intact. Morsellized bone is usually used for this type of defect.
2. *Minor Column (Shelf)*: Loss of part of the rim plus the corresponding acetabular wall but less than 50% of the acetabulum. A structural graft is used but less than half of the acetabulum is replaced. This is called a minor column or shelf graft.
3. *Major Column*: Loss of one or both columns with its corresponding acetabular wall involving over 50% of the acetabulum. A major column structural graft involving over 50% of the acetabulum is used.

## Surgical techniques

In our hospital, all revisions requiring the use of allograft bone are done in a laminar flow operating room with body exhaust systems. If there is preoperative evidence of infection or any suggestion at the time of surgery (even with a negative Gram's stain) the surgery is staged for any revision requiring the use of allograft bone.

Any allograft bone is brought into the operating room at the beginning of the case, unwrapped, cultured and immersed in warm Betadine. The bone is obtained from our own bone bank, where it has been deep frozen at −70°C after being irradiated with 2.5 megarads.

## Surgical approach

The surgical approach is either transgluteal[9], or trans-trochanteric. The trans-trochanteric approach is used most commonly because of the need for extensive exposure and also because in many cases there is a pre-existing trochanteric non-union.

The large fragment proximal femoral grafts should be done via the transtrochanteric approach and the trochanteric fragment should be kept as long as possible so that it will unite and reinforce the allograft. The proximal femur is exposed by reflecting the vastus lateralis off the septum anteriorly, being careful not to strip any residual bone of its soft tissue completely.

A Steinmann pin is inserted into the iliac crest as a reference point to adjust leg lengths. The distance from the pin to the rough line (insertion of the vastus lateralis) is recorded prior to dislocation.

## Acetabulum (Table 13.1)

The acetabulum is prepared after the hip has been dislocated. After the acetabular prosthesis and the cement are removed the membrane is excised carefully because of possible complete bony defects that instruments could penetrate through into the pelvis. The defect is then defined by visualization, palpation, and using a trial cup. At this point the defect must be defined so the allograft can be prepared. If the defect is a contained cavity (protrusio) then morsellized bone can be used. If the defect is a minor or major column defect, then a bulk allograft is indicated. If a bulk allograft can be avoided by raising the acetabulum 1 or 2 cm to get into better bone stock, then this alternative should be used because better contact with host bone is obtained[10] (Figure 13.1). Bulk allografts on the pelvic side should be

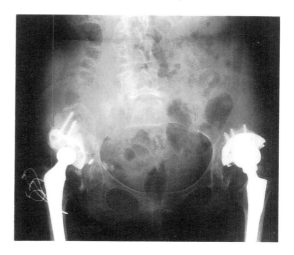

**Figure 13.1** High hip centre. A.P. X-ray of a 50-year-old female with bilateral revision arthroplasties. Both reconstructions have been placed high because she had adequate bone stock and leg length discrepancy was not a problem. This X-ray also demonstrates two methods for stabilizing the cup in a proximal location. The right hip was done with a reinforcement ring and a cemented cup and the left with an uncemented cup.

**Table 13.1 Summary of bone deficits and reconstruction for pelvis**

*SMALL DEFECT*

Autograft
Modified Implant

*LARGE DEFECT (Allograft)*

i. *Contained Cavitary Defect (Protrusio)*

    (a) *Low Demand Patient:* Morsellized bone and protrusio ring and cemented cup
    (b) *High Demand Patient:* Morsellized bone and large Diameter uncemented metal backed cup (porous coated press-fit or held with screws)

ii. *Structural Defect (Major or Minor Column Defect)*

    Minor Column – Uncemented or cemented cup (Shelf)
    Major Column – Cemented cup

avoided if possible and in the majority of cases, the acetabulum can be seated in host bone supplemented by morsellized allograft (protrusio graft). If a major or minor column defect does exist and cannot be compensated for by raising or centralizing the acetabular bed then a bulk allograft should be used. For bulk allografts we prefer to fashion true acetabular allografts but male femoral heads or even distal femurs can be used. If morsellized bone is used then female femoral heads should be used rather than sacrificing strong structural bone. We prefer not to use a bone mill because the bone is made too mushy. The bone can be easily morsellized by hand using curettes and rongeurs and is fine enough to pack into cavities but still has some structural integrity. Morsellized bone can be packed into cavities using the acetabular reamers in reverse.

Allograft bone can be further classified according to how it is used: (1) morsellized (2) structural: (a) simulated, (b) anatomical.

A simulated structural graft is where bone from another region is shaped to simulate the deficit. For example a distal femur can be sculpted to duplicate an acetabulum.

An anatomical structural graft is when the graft is the actual anatomical part being duplicated. For example an acetabular allograft is used in whole or in part to replace an acetabular defect.

The advantages of a structural graft are restoration of anatomy and they can provide structural support for the implant. The disadvantage of a structural graft is that revascularization and remodelling can lead to resorption and/or collapse and therefore weakens with time.

Structural grafts are indicated for uncontained defects where it is necessary to restore anatomy and leg length and to provide bone support for the implant. Acceptable compromises to the anatomy and leg lengths are preferable to structural grafts if adequate bone stock is available, i.e. high hip centre[1].

Morsellized bone is indicated for contained defects where it serves as a filler scaffold. It can undergo revascularization and remodelling and strengthens with time. It cannot be used for early structural support.

All reconstructions will eventually fail whether they are synthetic or biological. As surgeons, our role is to prolong the time to failure, and to make sure that when failure occurs further reconstruction

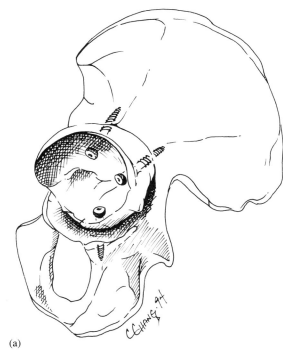

(a)

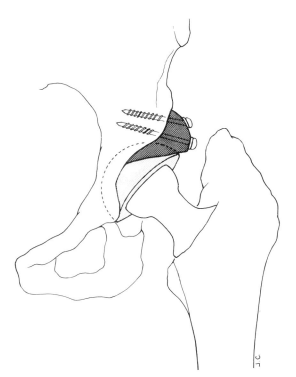

**Figure 13.2**  Drawing of minor column (shelf) reconstruction. The allograft is slotted into the deficit so that some host bone overlies the allograft. Fixation is provided by two oblique 4.5 mm cancellous screws. Autograft cancellous bone is placed between the allograft and the host ilium (flying buttress graft).

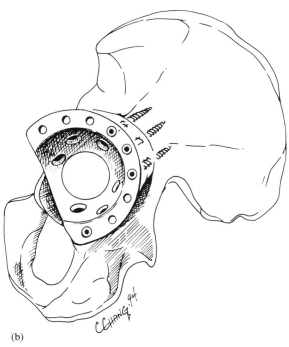

(b)

**Figure 13.3**  Drawing of major column reconstruction. a, Pelvic allograft held by large 6.5 mm cancellous screws prior to application of reinforcement ring. b, Pelvic allograft held by large cancellous screws and reinforcement ring to bridge graft from host bone to host bone.

is possible. Bone grafts restore bone for future surgery.

Minor column grafts can be fixed by two vertical to obliquely oriented cancellous screws (4.5 mm) (Figure 13.2). Reinforcement rings or reconstruction pelvic plates are used for the major column grafts (Figure 13.3). If possible it is our preference to bridge these major column grafts from host bone to host bone using a plate or a reinforcement ring. It is best not to ream these grafts, but if it is necessary, the cartilage is reamed off leaving the subchondral bone intact. It is done very lightly with the grafts fixed in position. If possible do not expose cancellous surfaces of the allograft to anything but host bone.

There are several options for the acetabular prosthesis. In the protrusio situation, morsellized bone, a reinforcement ring and a cemented cup is a good reconstruction for the moderate to low demand elderly patient (Figure 13.4). The best reconstruction for a protrusio defect in the higher demand patient is morsellized bone with an uncemented

fixed large diameter, metal backed porous coated cup with direct contact with at least 50% host bone (Figure 13.5). In most cases screws are necessary to fix the cup. Bipolar or biarticulating cups are only used if nothing else is technically or biologically possible, or because of the patients' health a more extensive procedure is not indicated.

A shelf or minor column defect will allow contact with at least 50% host bone and here we prefer to use an uncemented porous coated cup, press-fit or fixed by screws. A cemented cup may, however, be used (see Figure 13.2).

A major column graft involves more than 50% of the acetabulum which means the cup is mainly in contact with dead allograft bone. Under these circumstances, the cup should be cemented (see Figure 13.3).

We attempt to obtain fixation of the porous coated cups by press-fit antirotation lugs, if possible. If not we use screws to fix the metal backing in place. We have had no experience with screw-in cups.

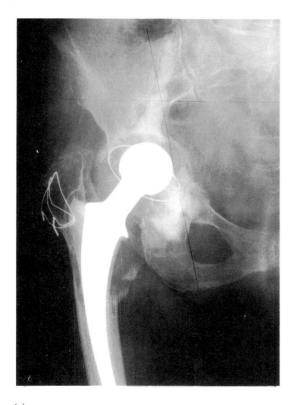

(a)

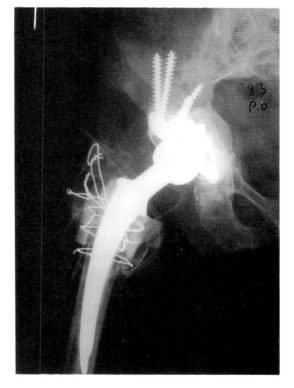

(b)

**Figure 13.4** Reconstruction of contained cavitary defect. a, A.P. X-ray left hip showing a contained cavitary defect and a loose acetabular component in a 70-year-old female.

b, A.P. X-ray left hip 6 years after reconstruction with morsellized allograft bone, a roof reinforcement ring and a cemented cup.

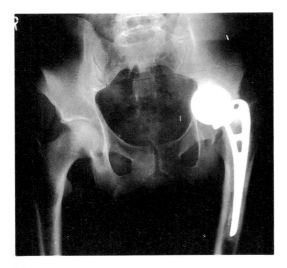

(a)

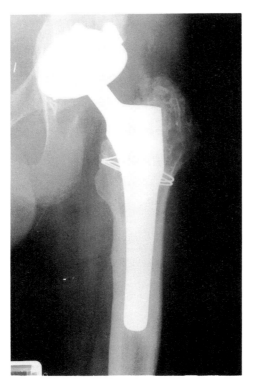

(b)

**Figure 13.5** Reconstruction of contained cavitary defect. a, A.P. X-ray 9 years after a Moore arthroplasty had been performed for osteonecrosis of the femoral head due to steroids. Migration of the implant has produced a superomedial protrusio. b, A.P. X-ray 7 years after reconstruction with morsellized allograft bone and a fixed large diameter uncemented cup.

Bipolar cups are only used in the extreme salvage situation where nothing else is possible for technical reasons, or because the patient's health will not tolerate a more extensive operative procedure (see Table 13.1).

## Postoperative care

Prophylactic intravenous antibiotics are used for 5 days followed by 5 more days of oral antibiotics. We prefer a cephalosporine. If the patient is catheterized intraoperatively, we use gentamicin during the surgery and for the first 24 hours but then switch to Septrin until the catheter is removed. Because of the extent of the surgery, we usually keep the patients on bed rest and in abduction for 5 days. The patients are not allowed any weight-bearing until union is obtained between allograft and host, usually at 3–6 months.

## Principles of surgery for acetabular grafting (see Table 13.1)

- Preoperatively decide on type of bone (morsellized or bulk), type of fixation and implant.
- Use an exposure that allows access to anterior and posterior columns. Trochanteric osteotomy is advantageous in most cases.
- Use internal fixation that goes from host bone to host bone if a structural graft involving over 50% of the acetabulum is used. Small grafts are fixed by cancellous screws oriented in an oblique to vertical direction.
- If a structural graft is necessary use strong bone, i.e. acetabular allograft, distal femur or male femoral head.
- If a structural graft involving over 50% of acetabulum is used cement the cup.
- Do not expose cancellous surface of graft to soft tissue of host if possible.
- Do not use structural grafts unless necessary (a) to provide support for implant, (b) to restore anatomy and leg lengths. Acceptable compromises to the anatomy and leg lengths are preferable to structural acetabular grafts if adequate bone stock is available, i.e. high hip centre.
- Autograft junction of allograft to host pelvis.

## Results

At 1 July, 1993, there has been acetabular revisions using morsellized allograft bone in 179 hips with an average follow-up of 4.57 years (range 1–11), 56 shelf grafts (minor column) with an average follow-up of 5.12 years (range 1–10), and 67 acetabular grafts (major column) with an average follow-up of 5.23 years (range 1–10).

A follow-up study of 58 reconstructions of contained cavitary defects using morsellized bone was carried out[4,11]. The follow-up average was 46.4 months (range 26–87). Morsellized allograft bone was used with an uncemented porous coated metal backed cup in 32 hips, with a Mueller ring and a cemented cup in 15 hips, and with a biarticulating device (bipolar) in 11 hips.

A modified Harris hip scoring system was used[12] (Table 9.2). Failure was defined as a postoperative increase in score of less than 20 points or the need for further surgery as a result of problems with the allograft.

A successful outcome was seen in 100% of reconstructions with the Müller ring and the cemented cup, and 94% of the reconstructions using the uncemented cup. Only 64% of the reconstructions using the biarticulating device were successful.

Radiographic review demonstrates probable loosening (circumferential lucent lines of more than 2 mm) in 57% and definite loosening (migration or change of orientation) in 14% of reconstructions using reinforcement rings (average follow-up, 63 months). Possible loosening was seen in 5% of the uncemented cups at an average follow-up of 39 months. Of the bicentric reconstructions, 57% showed significant migration and less satisfactory pain reduction. Overall, the average medial migration of the bicentric devices was 3.2 mm (range 0–10) and superior migration averaged 17.0 mm (range 0–60). The superior lateral corner of the obturator foramina served as landmarks utilizing horizontal and vertical lines from the centre of the femoral head to determine superior and medial migration (Figure 13.6). In contrast, cemented implants with reinforcement rings averaged 0.1 mm of medial migration (range –1 to +1) and 1.7 mm of superior migration (range –6 to +12). The fixed non-cemented implants averaged 0.9 mm of medial migration (range –3 to +4) and 1.1 mm of superior migration (range –9 to +9).

Remodelling and resorption of the morsellized graft were observed. The final width of the bone graft was noted to be diminished compared with the immediate postoperative width. Percentage resorption was 5.7% (range 0–27) in the cemented cups, 50.6% (range 17–100) in the bicentric devices and 26.4% (range 0–83) in the non-cemented cups.

A follow-up study of bulk (major and minor column) acetabular allografts was performed[4,13]. A modified Harris scoring system was used (Table 9.2).

The average preoperative hip score for the solid fragment acetabular group as a whole was 30 (range of 4–60). Five patients were confined preoperatively to a wheelchair. Postoperatively the hip score averaged 74, with a range of 55–98. Failure occurred in 10 patients (one patient bilaterally). There was 1 failure by score alone. Seven patients required additional surgery for major column acetabular allograft complications and 3 patients needed surgery for minor column (shelf) allograft complications. Of the 8 reoperated arthroplasties, 6 are now considered to have successful clinical scores, despite this setback.

In this study there were 19 patients with 22 shelf (minor column) reconstructions with a follow-up of mean of 40.8 months (range 29–68). The mean preoperative score was 31 and postoperative 72. Two grafts had complete graft resorption. Eight grafts showed a stress shielding type of resorption or remodelling in which the unloaded portion of the graft was resorbed. This affected the most lateral part of the graft and usually involved 3–7 mm.

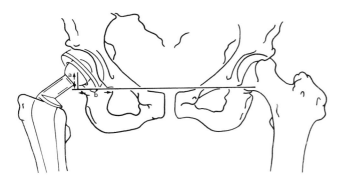

**Figure 13.6** Assessment of acetabular migration or protrusion after revision arthroplasty. The reference line is drawn through the superolateral corners of both obturator foramina. a = superior migration; b = medial migration.

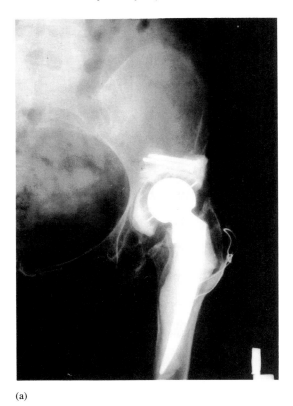

(a)

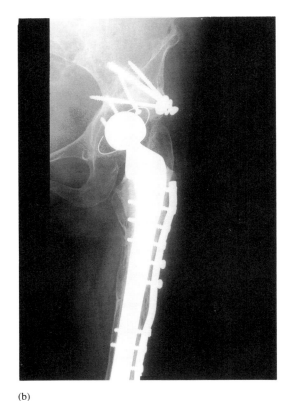

(b)

**Figure 13.7**   Minor column graft a, A.P. X-ray left hip of a 50-year-old female with failed loose cemented cup done for dysplasia. Bone graft was not used. b, A.P. X-ray 8 years after reconstruction with a minor column allograft and an uncemented cup.

Acetabular implant migration occurred in 3 cases, 2 of which were bipolar prostheses. Of the 22 shelf (minor column) grafts there were 3 failures, 2 for deep sepsis requiring further surgery, and 1 for a dislocated cup. The overall success rate was 86% (Figure 13.7).

In the major column group there were 28 reconstructions in 26 patients with a mean follow-up of 36 months (range 24–71). The mean preoperative score was 29, and the mean postoperative score 75.

There was 1 case of deep sepsis requiring excision in a reconstruction using femoral heads. A patient with flaccid paralysis (myelomeningocele) reconstructed with an acetabular allograft required further surgery for recurrent dislocation.

Six of the remaining 14 true acetabular allografts (i.e. reconstruction with acetabular allograft bone) required further surgery due to fracture or fragmentation of the graft. The subsequent reconstruction was greatly facilitated by the restored bone stock. Five of these 6 reoperated acetabular allografts have a successful clinical score 2 years after reoperation. The last patient with a bipolar reconstruction remains a failure due to the minimal increase in her clinical score after reoperation.

Six allografts were associated with implant migration and 5 of these cases involved a bipolar prosthesis that had eroded the allograft in varying amounts of 5–15 mm in a proximal medial direction. Only 1 of the 6 bipolar reconstructions was not associated with migration. The overall success rate for major column allografts was 71% (20 of 28 cases) (Figure 13.8).

A more recent review of our cases revealed the following data at 1 July, 1993:

Of 179 acetabular reconstructions using morsellized allograft bone, 9 have required revision (inc. 5%) at an average follow-up of 4.57 years. The reasons for revision were 4 cases for cup loosening and 5 for dislocation. All revisions were successful.

Of 56 minor column (shelf) allografts 4 revisions were necessary (inc. 7%) at an average follow-up of 5.12 years. Two were revised for loose

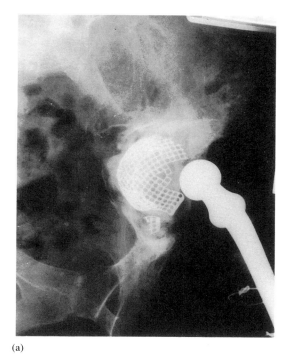

(a)

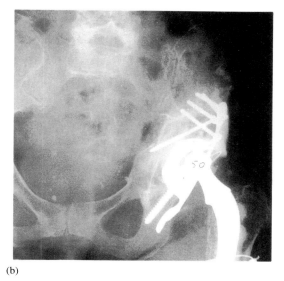

(b)

**Figure 13.8** Major column graft a, Judet view of left hip in a 40-year-old female showing severe loss of pelvic bone stock and a loose acetabular component. b, A.P. X-ray 10 years after reconstruction with major column allograft.

cups, 1 for infection and 1 for resorption. All were revised successfully.

Of 67 major column grafts 25 revisions in 16 hips have been necessary (inc. 37%) at an average follow-up of 5.23 years. Ten were revised successfully and 6 underwent excision arthroplasty. The reasons for revision or excision were as follows: dislocation 4 hips, loose cup 10 hips, non-union 5 hips, fracture 3 hips, infection 2 hips, and nerve injury 1 hip.

The incidence of revisions of major column grafts of 37% is inflated due to the fact that 16 hips had 25 complications (Figure 13.9). The incidence of patients requiring further surgery was therefore 16 of 60 = 27%.

**Figure 13.9** Major column graft — complication loose cup. a, A.P. X-ray pelvis of a 50-year-old female with right hip having been revised to a major column graft held by cancellous screws. The cup is cemented. The left hip was reconstructed with a minor column graft and an uncemented cup. b, A.P. X-ray 5 years later showing displaced cup. Although one screw is fractured allograft appears intact. c, A.P. X-ray after revision. The allograft was intact and solid. A new cup was cemented into a roof reinforcement ring which was also used to protect the allograft.

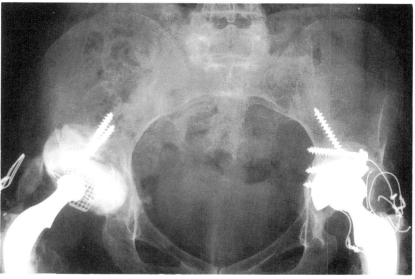

(a)

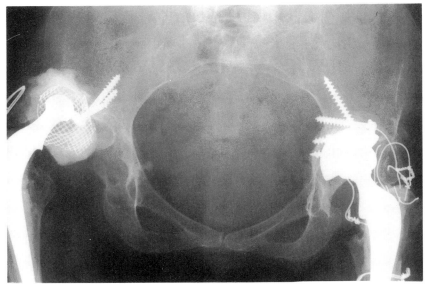

(b)

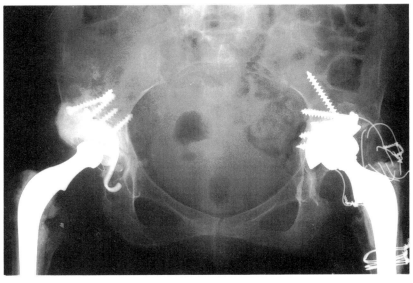

(c)

## Complications

At 1 July, 1993, in our entire group of revisions requiring allograft bone (384 hips in 357 patients), the following complications occurred. There were 26 dislocations (inc. 6.8%) with 18 requiring further surgery. There have been 10 infections (inc. 2.6%) with 3 requiring excision arthroplasty; 2 were revised and 5 left with a draining sinus. There have been 4 vascular complications including 1 intraoperative death. There have been 6 excision arthroplasties, 3 for infection, 1 for recurrent dislocation and 2 for displacement of pelvic allografts. There have been 5 nerve injuries with 3 recovering spontaneously, 1 requiring surgical repair, and 1 pending conservative treatment. There have been 5 deaths, 3 unrelated, 1 due to an intraoperative external iliac vein laceration and 1 due to intraoperative fat embolism. There has been 1 amputation for pain.

# References

1. Russotti, G.M. and Harris, W.H. (1991) Proximal placement of the acetabular component in total hip arthroplasty. A long-term follow-up study. *J. Bone Joint Surg.*, **73A**, 587–592.

2. Jasty, M. and Harris, W.H. (1990) Salvage total hip reconstruction in patients with major acetabular bone deficiency using structural femoral head allografts. *J. Bone Joint Surg.*, **72B**, 63.

3. Oakeshott, R.D., Morgan, D.A.F., Zukor, D.J. et al. (1987) Revision total hip arthroplasty with osseous allograft reconstruction. *Clin. Orthop.*, **225**, 37–61.

4. Gross, A.E. (1992) Revision arthroplasty of the hip using allograft bone. In *Allografts in Orthopaedic Practice* (A.A. Czitrom and A.E. Gross, eds) Baltimore: Williams & Wilkins, pp. 147–173.

5. Czitrom, A.A. (1992) Immunology of bone and cartilage allografts. In *Allografts in Orthopaedic Practice* (A.A. Czitrom and A.E. Gross, eds) Baltimore: Williams & Wilkins, pp. 15–25.

6. Langer, F., Czitrom A., Pritzker, K.P. et al. (1975) The immunogenicity of fresh and frozen allogeneic bone. *J. Bone Joint Surg.*, **57A**, 216.

7. Czitrom, A., Gross A., Langer, F. et al. (1988) Bone banks and allografts in community practice. *Instructional Course Lectures American Academy of Orthopaedic Surgeons*, **37**, 13–24.

8. Goldberg, V.M. and Stevenson, S. (1992) Biology of bone and cartilage allografts. In *Allografts in Orthopaedic Practice* (A.A. Czitrom and A.E. Gross, eds) Baltimore: Williams & Wilkins, pp. 1–13.

9. Hardinge, K. (1982) The direct lateral approach to the hip. *J. Bone Joint Surg.*, **64B**, 17–19.

10. Harris, W.H., Krushell, R.J. and Galanter, J.O. (1988) Results of cementless revisions of total hip arthroplasties using the Harris-Galante prosthesis. *Clin. Orthop.*, **235**, 120–126.

11. Allan, G.D., Butuk, D. and Gross A.E. (1991) Morsellized allograft reconstruction of contained cavitary defects in revision total hip arthroplasty. *Orthop. Trans.*, **15**, No. 3, 821.

12. Harris, W.H. (1960) Traumatic arthritis of the hip after dislocation and acetabular fractures: treatment by mold arthroplasty. An end result study using a new method of result evaluation. *J. Bone Joint Surg.*, **51A**, 737.

13. Gross, A.E., Allen, D.G. and Lavoie G.J. (1993) Revision arthroplasty using allograft bone. In *Instructional Course Lectures, Volume 42* (J.D. Heckman, ed.) American Academy of Orthopaedic Surgeons, Rosemont, pp. 363–380.

# 14

# Impaction grafting and cemented acetabular revision

Tom J.J.H. Slooff, Pieter Buma, Jan Willem Schimmel, B. Willem Schreurs, Jean Gardeniers and Rik Huiskes

## Introduction

In the period 1968 to 1989, 2461 primary total hip replacements of the cemented Müller curved stem design were performed and 471 replacements of the Müller straight stem design. From this series, a total of 261 total hip arthroplasties (=10%) were revised. In addition, a total of 149 revision arthroplasties were performed at our Institute which had initially been operated on at other clinics using a variety of prosthetic designs. We therefore performed 410 cemented revision procedures. Loosening of the acetabular components was associated with severe bone destruction in 134 cases. Since the mid-1970s, impaction grafting has been used to restore bone stock on the pelvic side and since the 1980s also on the femoral side, combined with cement fixation of the prosthetic component.

This chapter presents the history of the use of bone grafts in cemented revision total hip arthroplasty, an overview of our experimental investigations: the initial stability of the components in the grafted acetabulum and femur, the histology of graft incorporation and our clinical results after 10 years of application to the acetabulum. The principles, preoperative planning and surgical technique are also discussed.

## The history of the use of bone grafts in cemented revision total hip arthroplasty

Most of the graft incorporation data[1–18], obtained in the past, were related to animal experiments. This can be summarized as follows:

- The process of graft incorporation represents a sequence of events and reflects a partnership between graft and host-derived factors.
- The host contributes all the blood vessels and the cells required to incorporate the graft. The graft may serve as a scaffold to promote the host response, and the graft matrix stimulates cellular activity for bone formation from the host.
- Cortical grafts are incorporated slowly, unpredictably, irregularly, incompletely and with mechanical weakening. Compared to cortical grafts, cancellous grafts have a more open structure which, in theory, allows rapid vascular invasion and should therefore enable rapid, more complete and uniform incorporation.
- The incorporation mechanisms of solid and morsellized cancellous grafts are less clearly understood. The rigidity and size of a solid graft may stress-protect any new bone that is formed within it. It has been speculated that impaction of a chip graft leads to an increase in bone density and helps to prevent mechanical weakening.
- Irrespective of the type of graft, essential factors which influence the process of incorporation are the stability of fixation, the amount of contact, the vascularity of the host bone bed, the strain pattern and the degree of antigen-matching.

Based on this information, the clinical application of many types of graft should be considered for total hip arthroplasty revision. In the 1970s, Hastings and Parker[19] and Harris et al.[20] reported on acetabular reconstructions with bone chip wafers and solid corticocancellous bone grafts for primary and revision total hip arthroplasties, respectively. The grafts were combined with cement and metal reinforcement materials, such as meshes, screws and bolts. The indications for reconstruction were mainly pelvic protrusion and insufficiency of the acetabular roof and rim, caused by a primary idiopathic process or resulting from failed total hip arthroplasty. These initial reports were followed by clinical studies on patients with intrapelvic protrusion[21–23], using primary cemented arthroplasties combined with autogenous bone chips supported by a metal mesh.

In 1984 we published our experience with a modification of the techniques developed by Hastings[19] and McCollum[21], [24]. We used morsellized allografts and impacted the chips rigidly in the reconstructed acetabulum. In the case of segmental and cavitary defects, containment was made with metal meshes for the graft which resulted in direct stability of the reconstruction.

The technique of cement fixation and bone grafting has also been adopted by Hirst et al.[25], Olivier and Sanouiller[26], Berry and Mueller[27] and Rosson and Schatzker[28]. Depending on the severity of the acetabular defects, they combined this technique with the use of metal reinforcement materials, such as the Müller ring, the anti-protrusion cage and the Burch–Schneider cage.

The original technique described by Harris et al.[20] introduced the use of solid grafts but provided only a short-term solution. Recently Harris et al. have published arguments against the use of solid weight-bearing allografts[29–31].

In order to obtain more insight into the incorporation process of the graft and into the initial mechanical stability of acetabular and femoral reconstructions using impacted morsellized allografts, we performed two animal experiments.

# Animal experiments

Both the acetabular and femoral reconstruction techniques using impaction grafting and cement were developed and tested on animal models[32–37]. The animal of choice was the goat.

The aims of these experiments were to make:

A. Histological evaluation of the different processes involved in the incorporation of (1) acetabular and (2) femoral grafts and,
B. Mechanical evaluation of the initial stability (*in vitro*) and stability of cemented (1) acetabular and (2) femoral components after incorporation of the graft.

## Materials and method

All the trabecular bone grafts were harvested from the sternum of donor goats under sterile conditions. The grafts were freshly frozen and stored at –80°C ready for implantation. In adult goats, the right hip was operated on under general anaesthesia using standard aseptic techniques. A dorsolateral incision was used, followed by dislocation of the hip and resection of the femoral head. Acetabular and femoral reconstructions were performed in two separate animal experiments. After the operation all the goats were kept in a hammock for 2 days. AP and lateral radiographs were taken immediately after the operation. The goats were then kept in cages which allowed free walking or in a field.

### Surgical technique

The acetabular cartilage was removed and a cavitary defect was made in the anterosuperior segment of the acetabulum using hand reamers. Impaction grafting of the resulting defect was performed in the same way as during clinical application to patients. The acetabular component was cemented. Three specimens were used to analyse the initial stability (*in vitro*). Six goats were sacrificed at intervals of 6, 12, 24 and 48 weeks. Three of the 6 cases from each interval were used for histology and three for biomechanical analysis.

The surgical approach to the femur consisted of preparing the medullary cavity with hand reamers. A concentric intramedullary graft could be impacted in a retrograde fashion (Figure 14.1) using a specially developed set of instruments. Cement was inserted into this construction, followed by the insertion of the femoral stem. The clinical application of this technique to patients has recently been published[38, 39]. To evaluate the femoral reconstruction we used 18 goats. The initial stability of the reconstruction was analysed in 4 specimens *in vitro*. To evaluate the postoperative changes, 7 goats were sacrificed after 6 and 12 weeks. Four specimens from each period were used for the biomechanical study, the other 3 were used for histological analysis.

### Biomechanical method

For mechanical testing of the grafted acetabulum and femur, tantalum pellets were fixed to both components prior to insertion. The 3D displacement of the components relative to the bone

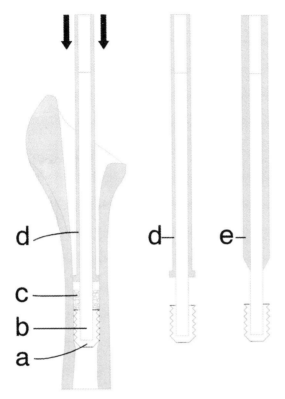

**Figure 14.1** Schematic representation of the graft impaction technique by using a special set of instruments. A bone cement plug (a) is screwed on a metal rod (b) and introduced into the canal. The space between this metal rod and the cortical bone is filled with trabecular bone grafts (c). These grafts are impacted using metal tubes sliding over the central rod. Different types of tubes are used for axial (d) and radial impaction (e) of the grafts (from Schreurs et al.[36]).

(rotation and translation) was measured using Röntgen-Stereophotogrammatic Analysis (RSA), developed by Selvik[40].

The acetabula and femora for the mechanical study were freshly harvested and stored at −80°C ready for testing. After thawing, both bone specimens were embedded in polymethylmethacrylate (PMMA). Tantalum pellets were inserted into small holes drilled into the pelvic and femoral bones in standard positions. Furthermore, small PMMA rods containing tantalum pellets were glued to the proximal, medial and lateral parts of the femoral prosthesis and inserted into the acetabular component. The prostheses–bone structures were then loaded into a MTS-testing device in a physiological way (Figure 14.2). A pelvic load was

applied stepwise from zero to 350 and to 700 N and again unloaded. Stereoröntgenograms were taken before loading, after each loading step and 10 minutes after the final unloading. A femoral load was also applied stepwise from zero to 200, 500, 800 N and again unloaded. Each loading period lasted 10 minutes.

All stereoröntgenograms were evaluated on an Aristomat digitizer, and the 3D pellet positions were determined with the RSA computer programme. Relative rotations and translations around and along the coordinate axes were calculated. To increase the accuracy of the results, all the stereoröntgenograms were measured 5 times and the results were averaged.

## Histological methods

The goats received different types of fluorochrome to enable the qualitative evaluation of bone ingrowth into the graft[41]. The acetabula and femora were harvested after perfusion of the lower extremity with Micropaque[R] as described by Rhineländer and Baragry[42]. After fixation in a buffered paraformaldehyde solution the acetabula and femora were contact-radiographed and sectioned with a water-cooled saw into slices of 2–3 mm. Radiographs were taken of the slices. Calcified and decalcified bone sections of various thickness were subsequently stained according to routine protocols.

## Histological evaluation of the grafted acetabulum (Figure 14.3)

The impacted graft consisted of fairly large pieces of trabecular bone, which displayed small microfractures at all levels. Generally, the bone graft was devoid of any well-preserved osteocytes, the osteocytes had completely resolved, or if they were still present, they had a very pyknotic appearance. Most of the medullary fat in the pieces of graft had been squeezed out during the process of impaction and had been replaced by a fibrin clot. Owing to surgical trauma, a circumferential necrotic zone of about 1–4 mm was found in the host bone. After revascularization of the host bone, a front of vascular sprouts accompanied by loose connective tissue with many macrophages, penetrated into the graft at a speed of about 70 µm per day. A very high dynamic bone turnover was observed in the graft in association with this granulation reaction, comprising bone graft resorption by osteoclasts and bone apposition by osteoblasts. This resulted

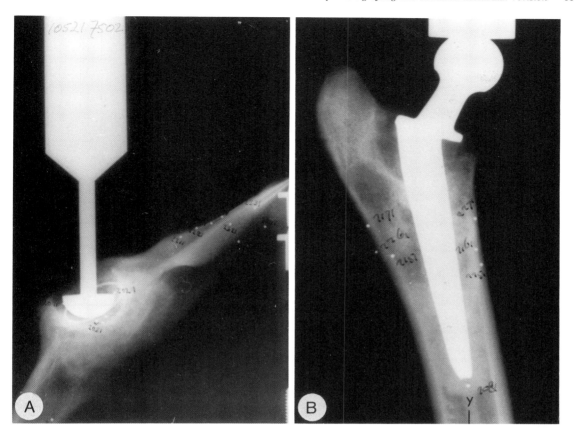

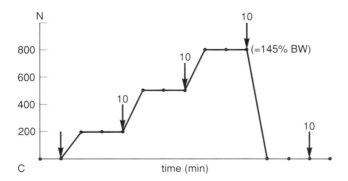

**Figure 14.2a,b**   Loading position of the acetabulum and femur in the MTS-machine. c, The loading schedule of the femoral intramedullary grafts. Stereoröntgenograms were made 1 and 10 minutes after each step in load (arrows).

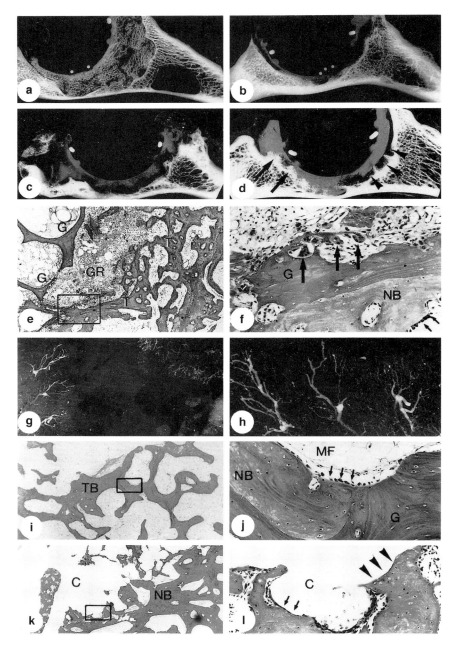

**Figure 14.3** Röntgenograms of thick sections through the acetabulum of the goat taken at 0 (a), 12 (b), 24 (c) and 48 weeks (d) after surgery. a, Note large pieces of graft and the clear transition zone to the host bone bed. b, Complete consolidation of the graft with the host bone. The incorporation of the graft is almost completed. c, A radio-lucent zone is present between the cement layer and the bone, indicating that a soft-tissue interface has been formed. d, Note local contact areas between bone and cement (arrows) and a radio-lucent zone (arrow heads). Note also the dense bone adjacent the cement layer. e, Granulation tissue (GR) in the transition zone between avital graft (G) and newly-formed trabecular bone (T) three weeks after surgery. f, Enlargement of encircled area in e. Many osteoclastic bone cells (large arrows) resorb the graft (G) and osteoblasts (small arrows) synthesize new bone (NB). g, A vascularization front penetrates into the graft (G) 12 weeks after the surgery. Cement (C) had penetrated into the graft. h, Enlargement of left part of g.i, Structure of new trabecular bone after 12 weeks. j, Enlargement of encircled area in i showing active osteoblasts (arrows) and new bone (NB). Remnants of the graft (G) can be recognized by the empty osteocyte lacunae. k, Interface between new bone (NB) and the cement 48 weeks after surgery. Cement (C) that was removed during processing of the tissues, had penetrated deeply into the graft. l, Locally at higher magnification a very thin, one cell layer thick (arrows) soft-tissue interface is present, while at other locations the new bone is in direct contact with the cement layer (arrowheads). e, g, i, k ×12.5; f, h, j ×125 (from Slooff et al.[43]).

in a new trabecular structure which consisted of a mixture of the remnants of the graft and newly-formed, mainly woven bone. Subsequently the percentage of graft in the new trabecular structure decreased further by bone remodelling. Radiographic and histological evaluation demonstrated that the orientation of the newly-formed trabecular bone was such that load transfer was possible from the cement layer to the host bone bed. After 12 weeks, the amount of bone graft was minimal and lamellar bone was found in the new structure. A fibrous tissue membrane of varying thickness had developed at the cement–graft interface. However, all the animals showed local areas where vital bone was in intimate contact with the cement layer, without the interposition of such a soft-tissue interface. Between 24 and 48 weeks after surgery, the graft in the defect of the acetabulum and femur had become completely revascularized. The percentage of graft present in the new bony structure was very low. Direct bone–cement contact sites were still present.

## Histological evaluation of the grafted femur (Figure 14.4)

In the femoral study the same observations were made. There was a clear difference in revascularization, consolidation, incorporation and remodelling of the graft between proximal levels where the graft was in direct contact with trabecular bone and more distal levels along the stem of the prosthesis where the graft was in contact with compact cortical bone. Cortical bone remodelling of the necrosis induced by disruption of the endosteal circulation, preceded the process of graft incorporation. Proximally, the process of revascularization took place much faster, which resulted in a difference of about 6 weeks in the incorporation process. Again bone resorption and new bone apposition on the graft resulted in a mixture of graft and new bone. As expected, there was more remodelling of the graft in the 12-week group and the remodelling process was not completed after 12 weeks, which was in accordance with the histological results of the acetabulum. Cement had penetrated into the graft to a depth of at least 1 mm. A soft-tissue interface (20–100 µm) was generally seen between the graft and cement, but again there was direct contact between the graft and cement at some sites with active bone formation in the direct vicinity of the cement mantle.

## Mechanical evaluation of the acetabulum (Figure 14.5)

All the specimens seemed to be firmly fixed when tested manually. Co-ordinate axes were chosen as follows: X axis dorsoventral, Y axis craniocaudal, Z axis medial–lateral. In most of the specimens, elastic recovery was observed after unloading. Initial stability was considered by testing the specimens immediately after implantation. Maximum persistent translation in this group was found in a craniocaudal direction (0.6 mm). Maximum rotation was measured around the X-axis ($-3.1°$). In course of time a rather consistent pattern was observed showing increasing stability after 12 weeks of implantation. Persistent translation in all directions declined from the zero group to the 12-week group, as was the case for rotations. At 12 weeks maximum persistent translation was measured in a medial–lateral direction (0.2 mm) with maximum persistent rotation around the Z axis ($-2.1°$).

## Mechanical evaluation of the femur (Figure 14.6)

In the *in vitro* study, which estimated the postoperative stability immediately after the operation, the most important motions were axial rotation and subsidence of the stem (max. 2.1°, and 0.500 mm, respectively). In the *in vivo* study, the maximum load on the femoral head (800N) was estimated to be at 145% of the body weight. The loading mode applied resulted in bending and rotational forces, which are important for testing the stability of hip prostheses. In agreement with Schreurs et al.[33], the stability after 6 and 12 weeks implantation had clearly increased relative to the initial stability of the stems immediately after insertion. In the 6 and 12 week specimens, most of the motion was axial rotation and subsidence and they both increased with increasing load. The maximum rotation was 0.24° under 800 N, but after unloading there was significant elastic recovery which resulted in a maximum permanent rotation of 0.14°. There were no differences between the 6 and 12 week groups. Maximum subsidence under a load of 800 N was 0.164 mm, while after unloading the maximum permanent subsidence was 0.078 mm. Although there were no significant differences between the results of the 6 and 12 week specimens, there was a trend towards greater permanent displacement in the 12-week group. The standard deviations for translations and rotations observed during biomechanical testing were estimated to be 0.036 mm and 0.07°, respectively.

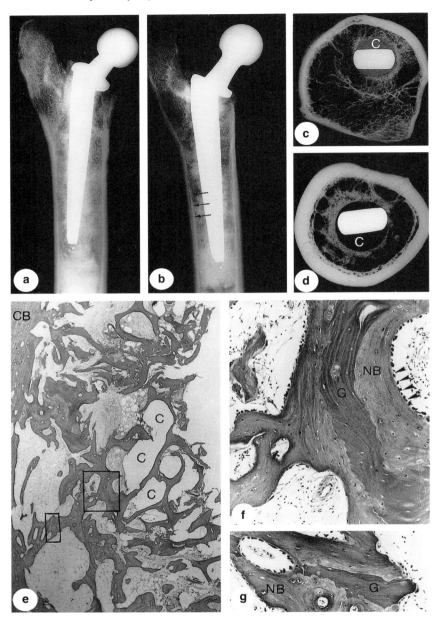

**Figure 14.4**   a and b, Röntgenograms of the prosthesis after 6 and 12 weeks, respectively. Note in a the change in trabecular appearance between the lateral proximal and more distal regions around the prothesis. b, Locally a radiolucent line is present in the cortical bone (arrows). c and d, Röntgenograms of thick sections of the proximal (c) and mid-shaft level (d) of the femur after 12 weeks. Note the orientation of the trabeculae from the cement layer (C) to the pre-existing cortical host bone. e, H & E stained section midshaft after 12 weeks. The graft is incorporated into a new bony structure that connects the cement layer (C) with the host cortical bone (CB). Note the penetration of the cement into the graft (×18). f and g, Enlargements of the boxed areas in e. Note that the trabeculae are a mixture of new bone (NB) and remnants of the graft (G). Osteoblasts (arrowheads) are present indicating bone formation, (×150) (from Schreurs et al.[36]).

## Conclusions from the animal experiment

The reconstruction technique resulted in rapid union between the graft and the host bone. From 12 weeks onwards, very little of the impacted bone graft remained. Instead a new trabecular bony structure of lamellar bone had formed. Although a fibrous tissue membrane of modest thickness had formed in some areas at the bone–cement interface, direct contact was present at some sites between the cement and newly-formed bone.

Our histological and mechanical results showed that the reconstruction technique provides sufficient initial stability to enable the incorporation of the impacted acetabular and femoral grafts.

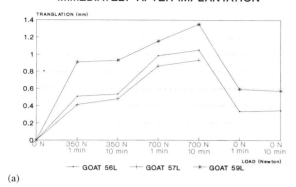

(a)

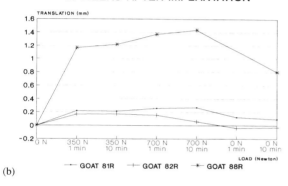

(b)

**Figure 14.5** Translations found in craniocaudal direction (Y axis) immediately after implantation (a) and after 12 weeks after implantation (b). Implant in goat 88R showed excessive translations and rotations in all directions and was considered loose.

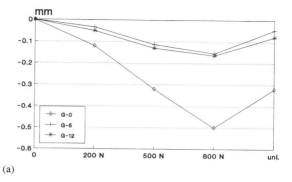

(a)

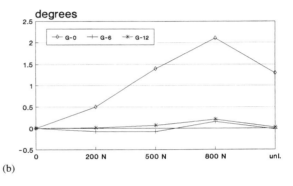

(b)

**Figure 14.6** a, Maximal femoral subsidence after 0, 6 and 12 weeks. Note increasing stability after incorporation of the graft. b, Maximal rotations of the graft after 0, 6 and 12 weeks showing the same trend.

## Principles for clinical application to the acetabulum

Although the follow-up period in the above-described animal experiments was limited to 48 weeks and the surgically prepared host bone bed was far less compromised than in human surgery, the results of the experimental study encouraged us to apply this biological reconstruction method to clinical acetabular[26, 44] and femoral deficiencies[38, 39]. The clinical instruments for the femoral technique were implemented and developed in close collaboration with Mr Ling and Mr Gie (from Exeter) and Howmedica International (Staines, England). Studies performed during the past few years have provided increasing support

for choosing the most appropriate approach to acetabular reconstruction[20, 26, 27, 29, 31, 43–51]

The aims of acetabular reconstruction are:

• restoring the centre of rotation
• restoring acetabular integrity
• providing adequate containment of the graft and socket
• achieving direct stability of the reconstruction

These aims were achieved by employing the following surgical measures (Figures 14.7, 14.8):

• Segmental defects were repaired with a wire mesh. In this way acetabular integrity was obtained which resulted in adequate containment of the graft.

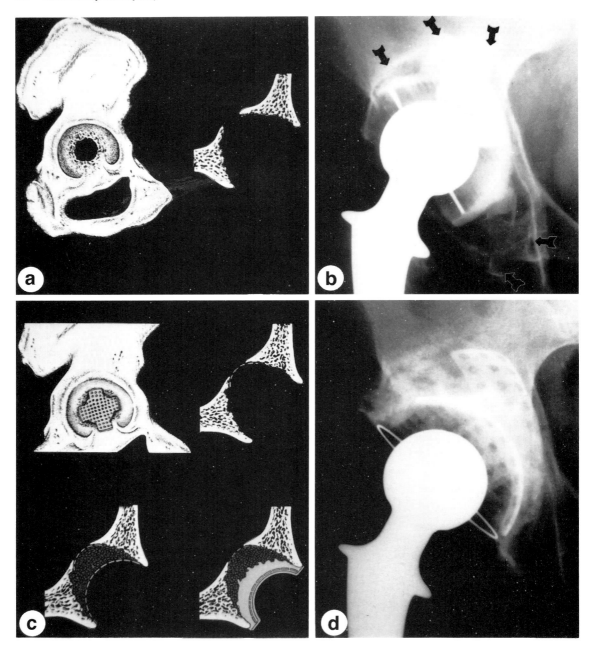

**Figure 14.7**   a, Schematic view of medial segmental defect. b, preoperative radiograph of medial segmental defect. c, Acetabular reconstruction of medial segmental defect. d, Radiograph 5 years after acetabular reconstruction with impaction grafting and cement (from Slooff et al.[43]).

- Cavitary defects were closed with wire mesh and augmented with tightly impacted morsellized cancellous allografts. As much graft material as necessary was packed until the trial socket was built up to the level of the transverse ligament, i.e. the anatomical location of the acetabulum. In this way, it was possible to use only conventional-size implants.
- After packing, the graft was covered with a flexible wire mesh to spread the load evenly over the graft.

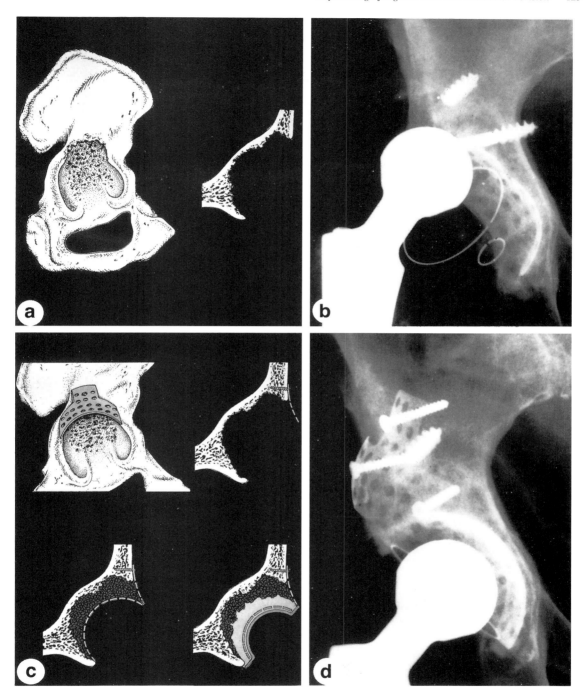

**Figure 14.8** a, Schematic view of combined segmental cavitary defect. b, Preoperative radiograph of a patient with a combined defect. c, Schematic view of reconstruction. d, Postoperative radiograph after cemented acetabular reconstruction with impaction grafting (from Slooff et al.[43]).

- Bone cement was used to stabilize the reconstruction directly. The hemispherical surface of the graft provided an ideal rough surface to interlock the cement.

Since 1978, this surgical technique for acetabular reconstruction has been standardized and is still being used today.

## Preoperative planning

Preoperatively, the patients were treated systematically according to a standard protocol. Our attention was chiefly directed at making the diagnosis of loosening and establishing the cause of failure. Once the diagnosis had been established, clinical treatment started with the direct or delayed exchange of components or resection arthroplasty. Our patient records showed that many of the patients with loosened components were functioning without any complaints of pain. The loosening process resulted in resorption of the bone bed and formed the major indication to revise the arthroplasty. It is therefore vital to evaluate all the patients with total hip arthroplasty periodically according to a standard protocol of routine investigations, to monitor postoperative complaints, problems with wound healing, function and to prevent extensive loss of bone stock in the case of loosening. At our clinic, follow-up was carried out after 3, 6, 12 weeks and after 6 months, and then periodically at yearly intervals. If any radiographic changes were observed, the follow-up interval was reduced as a means to prevent extensive bone loss.

Before revision of the loose component, the patients underwent a thorough physical examination, including hip mobility and gait. Weight-bearing on the affected side often resulted in a positive Trendelenburg sign. Reduction in the range of motion was rarely seen, but forced passive rotations were painful. A very reliable diagnosis of loosening could be made if the patient was unable to raise his/her leg while keeping it straight. Local examination of the hip and soft tissues was also important to locate previous incisions and areas of tenderness. Preoperatively, the neurovascular status and any discrepancies in leg length were assessed carefully. The thorough physical examination was followed by laboratory tests, including ESR, white blood cell counts and C-reactive protein. To assess loosening of the components, good quality plain radiographs were taken. These radiographs were used to evaluate the severity of the anatomical distortions, the location and extent of bone lysis, the distribution of cement, any deficiencies and bony defects. Serial radiographs were compared to monitor any progressive changes in the position of the component, the cement and the bone stock over the course of time. In this way, we were also able to detect very slowly progressing changes. The presence of a radiolucent line was not an indication of failure, but any radiolucency between the acrylic cement and bone which progressed in time, in extent and width, constituted a definite radiological and clinical diagnosis of loosening. Migration of the components and progressive bone destruction, which could be assessed easily on the serial radiographs if there was gross movement and abnormalities at the interface, reflected definite evidence of loosening. In cases of suspected loosening, preoperative management also included subtraction arthrography combined with an intra-articular needle biopsy and a bone scan to exclude septic loosening. Positive results and the exclusion of other causes of failure meant that the diagnosis of loosening was a distinct possibility.

## The standard operative technique

A posterolateral approach was used in all the cases and was combined with trochanteric osteotomy in only 3 cases. The proximal part of the femur was carefully released and mobilized, followed by dislocation of the hip. After testing for loosening, both components were released from the cement mantle. The whole socket of the acetabulum was exposed from the transverse ligament to the superior margin, and from the posterior wall to the anterior wall. After removing the socket and the cement, the fibrous interface was separated from the thin irregular acetabular wall using sharp spoons. Removal of this layer led finally to abundant bleeding of the sclerotic bone. At least three specimens were taken of the interfacial fibrous membrane for frozen section and culture. After this procedure, a prophylactic antibiotic regimen was started. The wall and floor of the cavity were examined to establish their integrity, the bone quality and to detect any defects. Reconstruction aimed to achieve adequate containment of the graft by closing the cavitary and peripheral segmental defects with a metal mesh. The cavitary defects were then filled with impacted chip grafts. Finally, the graft was covered by a second metal mesh and a polyethylene cup was cemented to it with a diameter 4 mm smaller than the mould itself.

# Postoperative treatment

Postoperative treatment comprised anticoagulation therapy for 3 months and systemic antibiotics for 24 hours. Indomethacin was administered for 7 days to prevent heterotopic ossification. Passive motion exercises were started after 24 hours, partial weight-bearing after 6 weeks, and full weight-bearing at 3 months p.o.

# The series of patients

Between January 1979 and January 1988, 91 revision hip arthroplasties (83 patients) were performed at our Institute using the above-described acetabular reconstruction technique with impaction grafting and cement. The original reasons for performing primary hip arthroplasty were primary osteoarthritis in 35 cases, secondary osteoarthritis due to congenital dysplasia, femoral head necrosis or trauma in 42 cases and rheumatoid arthritis in 11 cases. The initial arthroplasties comprised 5 femoral head prostheses, 13 double cup prostheses and 70 total hip replacements. In 8 cases, the reason for revision was septic loosening; the procedure was performed in two or more stages after debridement and local and systemic antibiotic treatment. The remaining revisions were necessary because of aseptic loosening. Morsellized autografts were used in 15 reconstructions, morsellized cancellous allografts from the hospital bone bank were used in 70 cases and a combination of these grafts was used in 3 cases. Patients were excluded from the follow-up study if the revision procedure was performed without bone grafts or a metal acetabular reinforcement ring had been used.

In the first half of 1990, all the patients eligible to take part in the study were invited for a clinical and radiographic examination by two of the authors (T.S., J.W.S.). Seven patients (7 hips) had died of causes not related to the revision procedure. One patient (1 hip) was lost to follow-up. The majority of patients had been followed-up routinely at yearly intervals, so it was possible to study the records and radiographs of their last visit. Finally, 88 hips (80 patients) entered the study with an average follow-up of 70 months (range 24–132 months). The average age at revision was 62 years (range 33–89 years).

# Classification of acetabular defects

It is important to define and classify acetabular defects in order to make a preoperative plan, to standardize terminology and to compare different reconstruction techniques. The American Academy of Orthopedic Surgeons (AAOS) Committee on the Hip, has proposed a practical classification system for acetabular deficiencies[52]. The system defines two basic categories: segmental and cavitary defects. A segmental defect is any complete loss of bone in the supporting hemisphere of the acetabulum, including the medial wall. Cavitary defects represent a volumetric loss of bony substance from the acetabular cavity, including the medial wall. Pelvic discontinuity is a defect across the anterior and posterior columns with total separation of the superior and inferior acetabulum. Using this AAOS classification, our group comprised 44 cavitary defects, 43 combined segmental/cavitary defects and 1 segmental defect.

# Clinical results

At the time of the study, 4 acetabular components had been re-revised because of recurrent infection in 2 cases, and aseptic loosening with migration in the other 2 cases. Clinical evaluation of the remaining 84 hips was based on the Harris hip score. The clinical result was considered to be excellent with a score of (i) 9–100 points, good with (ii) 81–90 points, fair with 70–80 points and poor with less than 70 points. The average score of our study group was 78 points (range 23–100). In 90% of the hips, the score was 80 points or more.

# Radiographic results

Radiographs were used to assess the following processes:

- incorporation which included consolidation
- migration and
- radiolucency

### Consolidation

Consolidation of the graft, i.e. union of the graft to the host bed, was defined as the presence of clearly delineated trabeculae crossing the graft–host junction. Consolidation was complete in all 88 hips.

Graft incorporation was assessed according to the criteria of Conn et al.[53] and was defined as: identical radiodensity of the graft and host bone, with a continuous trabecular pattern throughout. Eight acetabula showed incomplete graft incorporation. Two cups had remained stable during the follow-up period, 5 cups had migrated with partial graft resorption but were clinically asymptomatic and 1 cup had been re-revised because of progressive loosening.

### Migration

Migration of the cup was established after digitizing the serial radiographs. Reliable reproducible measurements could be performed on the monitor. The position of the socket was determined by the metal wire marker on the cup and was measured relative to Köhler's line and the tear drop line. The reliability of this method was estimated at 5 mm. The 5 cups with incomplete graft incorporation showed definite migration and were considered to be loose.

### Radiolucency

Radiolucency at the graft–cement interface was assessed according to the criteria of DeLee and Charnley[54]. Cups with continuous lucent lines of greater than 2 mm in all the segments were considered to be loose. One cup showed progressive continuous lucency with incomplete graft incorporation but an absence of any migration.

We defined failure as:

| | |
|---|---|
| re-revision | 4 cases |
| migration > 5mm | 5 cases |
| continuous lucency > 2mm | 1 case |
| | 10 cases (11.4%) |

In our series of 88 cup revisions, we had 10 failures of which two were due to recurrent infection (2.3%).

The primary aetiology of the aseptic loosened cup comprised 4 loosenings (11.4%) in the primary osteoarthritis group, 3 loosenings (7.1%) in the secondary osteoarthritis group and 1 (9%) in the rheumatoid arthritis group. Excluding the septic failures, the failure rate in the cavitary-type defect group did not differ significantly from that in the combined cavitary/segmental defect group: 9.1% and 9.3% respectively. This indicates that there was no difference in structural stability between the contained and non-contained acetabular defects reconstructed with impaction grafting and cement.

## Conclusions

The clinical use of bone grafts in cemented revision acetabular reconstruction is a well-accepted surgical procedure. We developed a surgical method for revision THA with impaction grafting and cement. The impacted graft was used to replace severe bone loss, to restore acetabular anatomical distortions to normal and to improve the cement interlock. This surgical method was based on an animal investigation in the goat in which the incorporation process and the initial stability of the reconstruction were measured and evaluated. The experimental results encouraged us to apply the surgical technique in clinical practice. The clinical and radiographic results of 10 years experience with this reconstruction technique justify its use.

### Acknowledgements

The authors wish to thank Miss Diny Versleyen for generously performing and preparing the histological sections for the animal experiments and Mrs M.L. Beenen for help in manuscript preparation.

### References

1. Albee, F.H. (1923) Fundamentals in bone transplantation. Experiences in three thousand bone grafts. *JAMA*, **81**, 1429–1432.
2. Axhausen, G. (1911) Arbeiten aus dem Gebiet der Knochenpathologie und Knochenchirurgie. 1. Kritische Bemerkungen und neue Beitrage zur freien Knochentransplantation. *Arch. Klin. Chir.*, **94**, 241–281.
3. Brooks, D.B. et al. (1963) Immunological factors in homogenous bone transplantation. IV. The effect of various methods of preparation and irradiation on antigenicity. *J. Bone Joint Surg.*, **45A**, 1617–1625.
4. Burwell, R.G. (1969) The fate of bone grafts. In *Recent Advances in Orthopaedics* (G.A. Apley, ed.). London: Churchill, pp. 115–207.
5. Campbell, C.J. (1953) Experimental study of the fate of bone grafts. *J. Bone Joint Surg.*, **35A**, 332–346.
6. Enneking, W.F. and Mindell, E.R. (1991) Observations on massive retrieved human allografts. *J. Bone Joint Surg.*, **73A**, 1123.
7. Friedländer, G.E. (1991) Bone allografts: the biological consequences of immunological events. *J. Bone Joint Surg.*, **73A**, 1119–1123.
8. Friedländer, G.E. (1987) Current concepts review on bone grafts. The basic science rationale for clinical applications. *J. Bone Joint Surg.*, **69A**, 780.
9. Goldberg, V.M., Powell, A., Shaffer, J.W. et al. (1989) The role of histocompatibility in bone allografting. In *Bone Transplantation* (M. Aebi and P. Regazzoni, eds). Berlin: Springer-Verlag, p. 126.
10. Goldberg, V.M. and Stevenson, S. (1987) Natural history of autografts and allografts. *Clin. Orthop.*, **225**, 7.

11. Greco, F., De Palma, U., Spechia, A. and Santucci, A. (1989) Biological aspects of repair osteogenesis in cortico-spongy homologous grafts. *Ital. J. Orthop. Traumatol.* **23**, 491.

12. Heiple, K.G., Chase, S.W. and Herndon, C.H. (1963) A comparative study of the healing process following different types of bone transplantation. *J. Bone Joint Surg.*, **45A**, 1593–1612.

13. Mankin, H.J. and Friedländer, G.E. (1989) Bone and cartilage allografts: physiological and immunological principles. In (H.P. Chandler and B.L. Penenberg, eds). *Bone Stock Deficiency in Total Hip Replacement* Thorofare, NJ: Slack Inc., Chapter 1.

14. Ottolenghi, C.E. (1972) Massive osteo and osteoarticular bone grafts. Technique and results of 62 cases. *Clin. Orthop.*, **87**, 156–164.

15. Scales, J.T. and Wright, K.W.J. (1983) Major bone and joint replacement using custom implants. In *Tumor Prosthesis for Bone and Joint Reconstruction, the Design and Application* (E.Y.S. Chao and I.C. Irin, eds). Stuttgart: Thieme Verlag, pp. 149–168.

16. Solomon, L. (1991) Bone grafts: Editorial. *J. Bone Joint Surg.*, **73B**, 706.

17. Stevenson, S., Xiao Qing, Li and Martin, B. (1991) The fate of cancellous and cortical bone after transplantation of fresh and frozen tissue-antigen-matched and mismatched osteochondral allografts in dogs. *J. Bone Joint Surg.*, **73A**, 1143–1157.

18. Wilson, P.D. (1951) Experience with the use of refrigerated homogenous bone. *J. Bone Joint Surg.*, **33B**, 301–315.

19. Hastings, D.E. and Parker, S.M. (1975) Protrusio acetabuli in rheumatoid arthritis. *Clin. Orthop.*, **108**, 76.

20. Harris, W.H., Crothers, O. and Oh, I. (1977) Total hip replacement and femoral head bone grafting for severe acetabular deficiency in adults. *J. Bone Joint Surg.*, **59A**, 752.

21. McCollum, D.E., Nunley, J.A. and Harrelson, J.M. (1980) Bone grafting in total hip replacement for acetabular protrusion. *J. Bone Joint Surg.*, **62A**, 1065.

22. Roffmann, M., Silberman, M. and Mendes, D. (1982) Stability and osteogenicity of bone coated with methylmethacrylate bone cement. *Acta Orthop. Scand.*, **53**, 5B.

23. Roffmann, M., Silberman, M. and Mendes, D. (1993) Incorporation of bone graft covered with methylmethacrylate into the autoacetabular wall. *Acta Orthop. Scand.*, **54**, 580.

24. Sloof, T.J., Van Horn, J., Lemmens, A. and Huiskes, R. (1984) Bone grafting for total hip replacement for acetabular protrusion. *Acta Orthop. Scand.*, **55**, 593.

25. Hirst, P., Esser, M., Murphy, J.C. and Hardinge, K. (1987) Bone grafting for protrusio acetabuli during total hip replacement. *J. Bone Joint Surg.*, **69B**, 229.

26. Olivier, H. and Sanouiller, J.L. (1991) Acetabular reconstruction with cancellous bone grafts for revision of total hip arthroplasties. *French J. orthop. Surg.*, **5**, 2, 187.

27. Berry, D.J. and Mueller, M. (1992) Revision arthroplasty using an anti-protrusio cage for massive acetabular bone deficiency. *J. Bone Joint Surg.*, **74B**, 711.

28. Rosson, J. and Schatzker, J. (1992) The use of reinforcement rings to reconstruct deficient acetabula. *J. Bone Joint Surg.*, **74B**, 716.

29. Harris, W.H. (1993) Management of the deficient acetabulum using cementless fixation without bone grafting. *Orthop. Clin. North Am.*, **24**, 663–665.

30. Kwong, L.M., Jasty, M. and Harris, W.H. (1996) High failure rate of bulk femoral head allograft in total hip acetabular reconstructions at ten years. *J. Arthroplasty*, (in press).

31. Mulroy, R.D. and Harris, W.H. (1990) Failure of acetabular autogenous grafts in total hip arthroplasty. *J. Bone Joint Surg.*, **72A**, 1536.

32. Buma, P., Schreurs, B.W., Versleyen, D. et al. (1992) Histologic evaluation of allograft incorporation after cemented and non-cemented hip arthroplasty in the goat. In *Bone Implant Grafting* (J. Older, ed.). London: Springer Verlag, p. 12.

33. Schreurs, B.W., Huiskes, R. and Slooff, T.J.J.H. (1990) The initial stability of hip prostheses in combination with femoral intramedullary bone grafts. Proceedings 7th Meeting European Society of Biomechanics, Aarhus, DK, A14.

34. Schreurs, W., Huiskes, R., Sloof, T.J.J.H. and Buma, P. (1992) A method to estimate the initial stability of cemented and non-cemented hip stems fixated with a bone grafting technique. In *Bone Impant Grafting* (J. Older, ed.). Berlin: Springer Verlag, pp. 131–134.

35. Schreurs, B.W., Buma, P., Huiskes, R. et al. (1993) The initial stability of cemented and non-cemented femoral stems fixated with a bone grafting technique. Transactions ORS, 452, San Francisco, USA.

36. Schreurs, B.W., Buma, P., Huiskes, R., et al. (1994) Morsellized allograft for fixation of the hip prosthesis femoral component. A mechanical and histological study. *Acta Orthop. Scand.*, **65**, 267–275.

37. Schreurs, B.W., Huiskes, R. and Sloof, T.J.J.H. (1994) The initial stability of cemented and noncemented femoral stems fixated with a bone grafting technique. *Clin. Mater.* **16**, 105–110.

38. Gie, G.A., Linder, L., Ling, R.S.M., et al. (1993) Impacted cancellous allograft and cement for revision total hip arthroplasty. *J. Bone Joint Surg.*, **75B**, 14–21.

39. Gie, G.A., Linder, L., Ling, R.M.S. et al. (1993) Contained morcellized allograft in revision total hip arthroplasty. *Orthop. Clin. North Am.*, **24**, 717–724.

40. Selvic, G. (1974) A röntgen-stereophotogrammatic method for the study of the kinematics of the skeletal system. Thesis, University of Lund, Lund, Sweden.

41. Rahn, B.A. and Perren, S.M. (1971) Xylenol orange, a fluorochrome useful in polychrome sequential labeling of calcified tissue. *Stain Technol.*, **46**, 125.

42. Rhineländer, F.W. and Baragry, R.A. (1962) Microangiography in bone healing. Undisplaced closed fractures. *J. Bone Joint Surg.*, **44A**, 1273.

43. Sloof, T.J.J.H., Schimmel, J.W. and Buma, P. (1993) Cemented fixation with bone grafts. *Orthop. Clin. North Am.*, **24** 667–677.

44. Sloof, T.J.J.H. (1992) Acebular augmentation in cemented arthroplasty: pre-operative assessment and surgical technique. In *Bone Implant Grafting* (J. Older, ed.) Berlin: Springer Verlag, pp. 51–55.

45. Gross, A.E., Lavoie, M.V., McDermot, P. and Marks, P. (1985) The use of allograft bone in revision of total hip arthroplasty. *Clin. Orthop.*, **197**, 115.

46. Harris, W.H. (1982) Allografting in total hip arthroplasty; in adults with severe acetabular deficiency including a surgical technique for bolting the graft to the ilium. *Clin. Orthop.*, **162**, 150.

47. Jasty, M. and Harris W.H. (1990) Salvage total hip reconstruction in patients with major acetabular deficiency using structural femoral head allografts. *J. Bone Joint Surg.*, **72B**, 63.

48. Jasty, M. and Harris, W.H. (1988) Results of total hip reconstruction using acetabular mesh in patients with central acetabular deficiency. *Clin. Orthop.* **237**, 142.

49. Jasty, M. and Harris, W.H. (1988) Total hip reconstruction using frozen femoral head allografts in patients
with acetabular bone loss. *Orthop. Clin. North Am.*, **18**,
291.
50. Samuelson, K.M., Freeman, M.A.R., Levak, B. et al. (1988)
Homograft bone in revision acetabular arthroplasty. *J. Bone
Joint Surg*, **70B**, 367.
51. Trancik, T.M., Stuhlberg, B.N., Wilde, A.H. and Feilzlin,
D.H. (1986) Allograft reconstruction of the acetabulum during revision total hip arthroplasty. *J. Bone Joint Surg.*, **68A**,
527.
52. D'Antonio, J.A., Capello, W.N., Borden, L.S. et al. (1989)
Classification and management of acetabular abnormalities
in total hip arthroplasty. *Clin. Orthop.*, **243**, 126.
53. Conn, R.A., Peterson, L.F.A., Stauffer, R.N. et al. (1985)
Management of acetabular deficiency: long-term results of
bone grafting the acetabulum in total hip arthroplasty.
*Orthop. Trans.*, **9**, 451.
54. DeLee, J.G. and Charnley, J. (1976) Radiological demarcation of cemented sockets in total hip replacement. *Clin.
Orthop.*, **121**, 20.

# 15

# The future

Richard N. Villar

This book cannot pretend to have covered every aspect of revision surgery. However, it is a sign of the complexity of the situation that it has had to be written at all. Revision surgery is demanding practice, with developments appearing almost monthly in the orthopaedic literature.

What of the future, so difficult to predict? One imagines that in several decades' time our descendants will look back at joint replacement as a rather archaic activity. 'How could you have done that?' they might say. Biological resurfacing, or even simple medication, may be all that is required to reinstate normal hip function, as a better understanding of the causes of degenerative disease becomes apparent.

However, today's joint replacements *will* fail in time. Whatever supposed cure may or may not be found for osteoarthritis, an enormous revision load still awaits the orthopaedic profession. So many countries are struggling hard to increase the numbers of joint replacements performed, in the knowledge that demand is unstoppable. Government ideology does not always take into account the fact that hip replacement is an operation with a finite shelf life. For some countries in the world, hip replacement has yet to arrive. They, too, will be faced with a massive revision problem when their turn comes.

Revision surgery has advanced significantly in the past five years. Particularly so in the field of surgical instrumentation. No longer has the revision operation been relegated to the ranks of the impossible procedure, left for the trainee to undertake, alone, on a dark winter's night. It is now seen very much as a specialist operation. Cement removal has been made simpler with the develop-

ment of specific instruments, and devices such as ultrasound. The future will undoubtedly see greater development in this area.

Loss of bone stock can no longer be ignored, whilst at the same time supplies of allograft bone are limited. The general public are now fully aware of the dangers of transmissible disease, and would prefer not to receive allograft tissue unless unavoidable. The use of bone substitutes, despite their expense, is thus likely to become more widespread. Possibly also, external treatments will be devised that allow bone reconstitution without surgery being required. Genetic manipulation of other animal species may be a fruitful source of xenograft tissue, particularly if the genotype can be adjusted to approximate that of man.

One might hope that the percentage of patients coming to revision might decrease over the years to come. This may possibly be so as the primary procedure becomes more standardized. Most now realize the importance of regular follow-up of patients, so it is less likely that grossly substandard prostheses will survive for long in the marketplace. The importance of minimizing wear debris production is now established and further efforts are likely to be made to reduce such production still further with developments in biomaterials. Revision surgery may become technically easier if primary cementless designs can be seen to surpass the performance of established cemented replacements. This may become possible by the coating of the components with 'bone-friendly' materials. Hydroxyapatite is a good example of this.

But is revision surgery worthwhile doing at all? One might argue that quality of life improvement is not sufficient to justify the effort expended. But this would not be true. Long, arduous surgery it may be, but quality of life improvement can equal that of primary replacement, though perhaps for not as long. It is thus essential that maximum efforts are made to develop further this exciting area of orthopaedic surgery.

# Index

.